THIS BOOK IS DEDICATED TO:

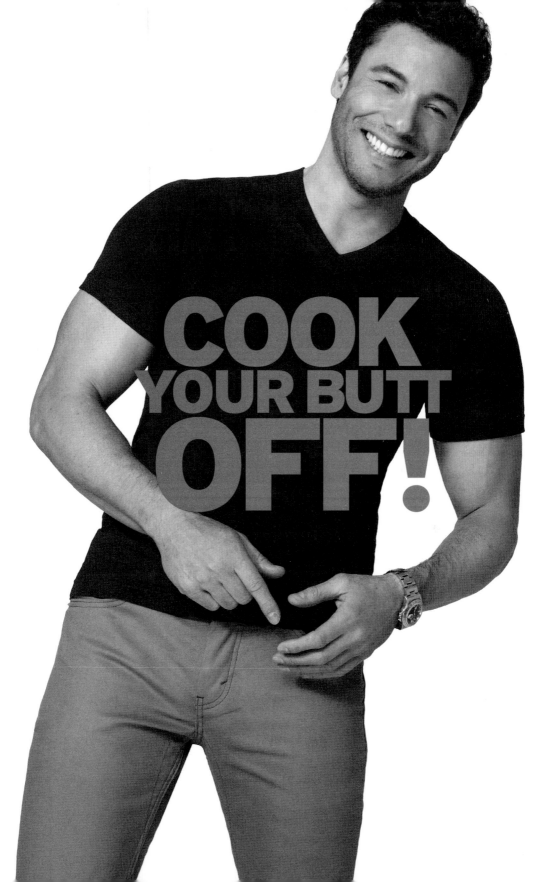

ALSO BY
ROCCO DISPIRITO

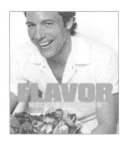

FLAVOR

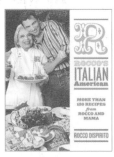

ROCCO'S ITALIAN-AMERICAN

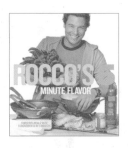

ROCCO'S FIVE MINUTE FLAVOR:
Fabulous Meals with 5 Ingredients in 5 Minutes

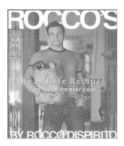

ROCCO'S REAL LIFE RECIPES:
Fast Flavor for Everyday

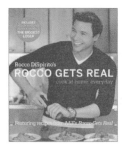

ROCCO GETS REAL:
Cook at Home Every Day

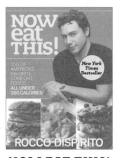

NOW EAT THIS!:
150 of America's Favorite Comfort Foods, All Under 350 Calories

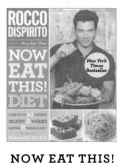

NOW EAT THIS! DIET:
Lose Up to 10 Pounds in Just 2 Weeks Eating 6 Meals a Day!

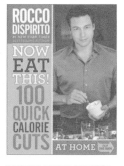

NOW EAT THIS! 100 QUICK CALORIE CUTS:
At Home/On-the-Go

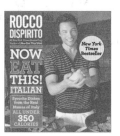

NOW EAT THIS! ITALIAN:
Favorite Dishes from the Real Mamas of Italy—All Under 350 Calories

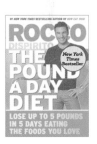

THE POUND A DAY DIET
Lose Up to 5 Pounds in 5 Days Eating the Foods You Love

COOK YOUR BUTT OFF!

LOSE UP TO A POUND A DAY WITH FAT-BURNING FOODS AND GLUTEN-FREE RECIPES

ROCCO DISPIRITO

GRAND CENTRAL
L&S
LIFE & STYLE

NEW YORK   BOSTON

Copyright © 2015 by Flavorworks, Inc.
Illustrations by Hsu + Associates

Grand Central Life & Style
Hachette Book Group
1290 Avenue of the Americas
New York, NY 10104
www.GrandCentralLifeandStyle.com

Design by HSU + ASSOCIATES

Printed in the United States of America

Q-MA

First Edition: February 2015

10 9 8 7 6 5 4 3 2 1

Grand Central Life & Style is an imprint of Grand Central Publishing.

The Grand Central Life & Style name and logo are trademarks of Hachette Book Group, Inc.

The Hachette Speakers Bureau provides a wide range of authors for speaking events. To find out more, go to www.HachetteSpeakersBureau.com or call (866) 376-6591.

The publisher is not responsible for websites (or their content) that are not owned by the publisher.

Library of Congress Cataloging-in-Publication Data

DiSpirito, Rocco

Cook your butt off! : lose upto a pound a day with fat-burning foods and gluten-free recipes / Rocco DiSpirito.

pages cm

Includes bibliographical references and index.

ISBN 978-1-4555-8352-2 (hardcover) — ISBN 978-1-4555-2370-2 (ebook) 1. Gluten-free diet—Recipes. 2. Reducing diets—Recipes. I. Title.

RM237.86.D57 2014

641.5'638--dc23

2014015981

CONTENTS

RECIPE INDEX

INSTRUCTION

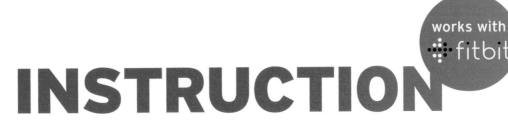

Why did I integrate Fitbit into this book?

I love activity trackers, and I wear my Fitbit every day. So do my clients.

Fitbit's devices track everything from steps taken, distance traveled, calories burned, active minutes to floors climbed, sleep quality, and heart rate! And the app just adds to the experience, by letting you record workouts, log calories, see your progress, and more.

For my clients, I use that information to tailor their menus to their individual weight loss goals. For myself, I use it to monitor my steps and calorie burn.

You don't need an activity tracker to use this book, but since Fitbit has been a great way for my clients and I to stay on track and meet our weight loss goals, I wanted to work with them to get all of the *Cook Your Butt Off!* recipes in their database of 350,000+ foods.

On each recipe page you'll see a Fitbit barcode. Simply scan it with the Fitbit app, and the calories and nutritional data will be automatically logged to your private Fitbit account.

And, if you're using a Fitbit tracker while you cook, you'll see how many calories you burn as you create each recipe—proving that you're really *cooking your butt off!*

> As of the date of publication, Rocco DiSpirito is a celebrity spokesperson for Fitbit.

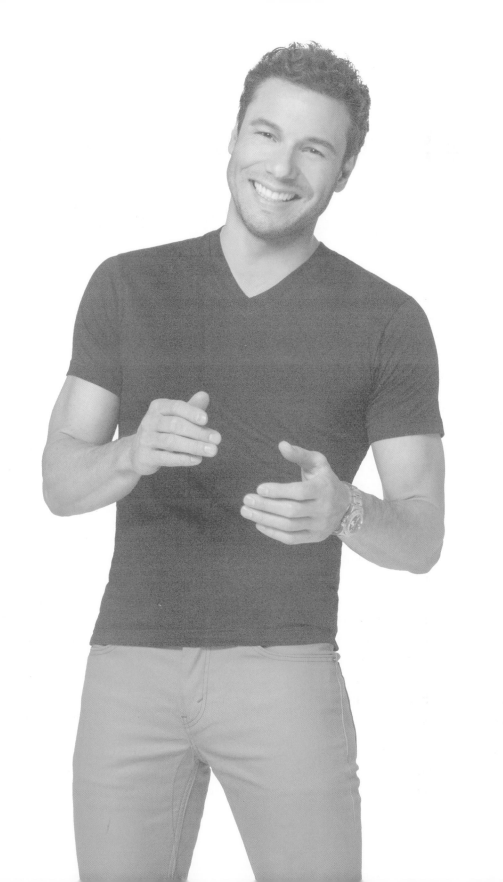

INTRODUCTION
Cooking—and Eating—for Life

I'VE spent the last several years devoted to healthy cooking that tastes amazing and helps you get lean and stay fit. I believe that everyone should be able to eat well, enjoy their food, and experience the physical and mental benefits that flow from this lifestyle. That is why I write the books I write and do the work I do.

For me, cooking is a passion and an integral part of who I am and where I come from. I am Italian, and we take cooking very seriously! As a small child, I would sit at my Nona's kitchen table in her home in West Hempstead, New York—a home, incidentally, where she completely re-created her Italian life—and she'd make me a simple but delicious egg dish with farm-fresh eggs, garlic, onions, peppers, and olive oil. That dish changed my life because it turned me on to the pleasures of cooking and serving good food—my life's work.

Decades later, as a professional chef, I was constantly surrounded by food. I was no longer in my Nona's homey kitchen but in full-blown restaurant kitchens, where the stress boiled over more frequently than the pots on the stovetop. Of course, it took its toll on my health. There are few days off in the food world and the breakneck pace of a busy restaurant is beyond demanding. As a whole, we chefs are not the world's healthiest eaters. As for following a particular diet—even one designed to make us feel better and lose weight—how could we be expected to do that? Day and night, we're tempted by incredibly delicious foods, which demand tasting at every stage. As for regular exercise, our long hours make it hard to squeeze in workouts beyond gathering up ingredients, chopping, mixing, stirring, standing at the stove, and pacing around the kitchen waiting for the dish to be done. (Turns out that cooking *can* be a workout, as you're about to see—but more on that later!)

About ten years ago, I was thirty pounds overweight, with an unhealthy 20 percent body fat, elevated blood pressure, and cholesterol. When a doctor asked me to draw up a will on the spot, only half-kidding, I knew I needed to make some serious changes. Cooking remained my passion, but now I had to find a new way to approach the foods I loved, because based on the doc's numbers, they had become the foods that were killing me.

I got back to a healthy weight and to better health by learning how to tweak recipes into lower-calorie, lower-fat versions of their former selves. I began to aggressively tinker with classic comfort food recipes and figure out how to downsize them in terms of calories, fat, and sugar, without sacrificing flavor or food quality. Think fried chicken, pizza, macaroni and cheese, and chocolate ice cream. I came up with versions of all those foods and many more—I called them the "bad boys" but I made them good, and good for you—in my bestselling NOW EAT THIS! books. I remain intent on finding more and more ways for eaters (myself included!) to enjoy lean, healthy makeovers of just about every favorite food, and to lose weight in the process. Yes, you can eat your favorite foods if you prepare them using the right techniques and recipes, *and* you can drop pounds. My last book, *The Pound a Day Diet*, has helped thousands do just that!

You could say that healthy food has become my vice—and I can't stop when it comes to coming up with new and improved versions of old favorites, taking out calories and adding in fabulous flavors, giving you recipes and techniques for turning out great-tasting food that will help you lose weight. Now I've created a new plan that will have you feeling better than ever in just two weeks. But these recipes aren't just reduced-calorie makeovers of foods you love; they are gluten-free, lactose-free, and totally free of refined sugar. As a result, they're naturally low in calories to help you drop pounds faster than ever. Even better, these recipes are free of ingredients such as gluten, lactose, and refined sugar that trigger allergies, upset your digestion, cause inflammation—and mess with your metabolism so that you pack on fat.

But there's one more secret weapon I'll reveal in a moment that ups the ante—and lowers the number on your scale. Let's just say that you'll be burning to cook these great-tasting foods! Read on and get ready to *Cook Your Butt Off!*

EAT THIS WAY NOW! (HERE'S WHY)

I love the way I feel now that I'm at a healthy weight and that I take better care of my body through regular exercise. My healthier lifestyle has come with an added bonus: I am more aware than ever of good nutrition through food, and I'm committed to encouraging others to eat well, too. Though my interest in nutrition grew out of concerns for my own health, along the way I became more knowledgeable about the topic—and more aware of the impact that poor eating habits have on our bodies. In fact, the horrifying health statistics of kids and adults in this country are what mobilized me to write the book you are now holding in your hands.

NOW READ THIS:

Kids today are eating themselves into an early grave. Consider: 17 percent of children and teens ages two to nineteen are obese (not just overweight, but downright fat), according to the Centers for Disease Control. Given that alarming rise in childhood obesity, it's estimated that more than one-third of all kids born in 2000 will eventually develop diabetes, either during childhood or when they hit their teen years.

And overweight five-year-olds are more likely to be obese by age fourteen than kids who began kindergarten at a healthy weight. This data comes from the Early Childhood Longitudinal Study conducted by the U.S. National Center for Education Statistics.

Who's to blame? Parents, schools, food manufacturers, society as a whole. If you ask me, making kids sick and fat is just another form of physical abuse.

I'll concede that life is tougher these days. In a time of single-parent and three-job families, people don't know how to cook anymore, or at the very least, they're pressed for time and resort to microwaveable processed foods or fat-laden fast foods and takeout. Somewhere along the line, too many of us have forgotten how to prepare fresh foods for ourselves and our families. It's quicker to zap a prepackaged meal or some snacks than make them from scratch—and kids are getting hooked on these lethal, chemical-filled foods. Unless we change our habits, and those of our children, the current generation could be the first to die younger than their parents.

Consider some other sobering statistics, all of which should serve as a wake-up call:

- *More than one-third of American adults are obese.*
- *Obesity-related conditions are sharply rising and include heart disease, stroke, type 2 diabetes, and certain types of cancer. These are some of the leading causes of* preventable *death.*
- *At the same time, millions of American families and children, or almost 15 percent of our households, experienced food insecurity during 2011, having no idea where they'd get meals for the week, and our food pantries are overwhelmed.*

None of this made sense to me: Our health-care system is the largest in the world, and we spend more money on our health care than the entire GDP of France, yet we are the world's most obese nation and more people die of obesity and obesity-related illnesses than all other illnesses combined.

Thanks to factory farming, we produce more food in calories than we need to consume as a nation. The average American consumes two times more calories than a body needs on a daily basis, yet 60 million Americans go hungry every day. The irony is that we're supposed to be the richest country in the world, and we produce the most food—but we can't feed our own people!

I am a strong proponent of healthy foods and good nutrition, and I find it difficult to reconcile the fact of the alarming obesity rate in this country with the data showing that there are so many hungry people. In this day and age, in this country, no one should have to go hungry.

I can't help reacting to these statistics. They've forced me to become a food activist, in addition to a chef and author. I've testified in front of Congress on the need to serve more nutritious food in school cafeterias and food banks, expand nutrition education and instruction, and address the unrighteous hunger problem in this nation. I've helped run food pantries to lend a hand to families facing food insecurity. I have a food truck on the streets of New York that serves fresh, low-calorie food and visits public schools to educate children on healthy eating, sustainability, and food security. And lately, I've been on a crusade to inspire people to buy locally grown, toxin-free foods. Doing so makes for a better way of life for everyone involved—from the people who raise and grow our food, to us, when we sit down at the table and enjoy what nature provides.

A NATURAL EVOLUTION: A MATTER OF TASTE AND HEALTH

I love the superior quality and taste of organic produce, and pasture-fed, responsibly raised meats. Most of all, I love the feeling of supporting small growers and farmers, particularly local producers. When I support the food producers in my area, I'm supporting people in my own community, and I'm preparing and eating foods that are good for my body and my weight. It's a win-win!

After I began eating more naturally, I started feeling like I could think more clearly, and I discovered the importance of maintaining my own well-being. If you don't know what you're putting in your body, you can develop some pretty serious problems, including chronic and even life-threatening illnesses. I learned that the hard way firsthand, when I was consuming too much of the wrong food. I cut back on fat, but I also took it a step further and started to reduce and even eliminate potential troublemakers like gluten, lactose, and refined sugar.

I felt even better—and really managed to keep the weight off. I changed what I put into my grocery cart because it was good for the environment and for my health, and now I'm going to teach you how to do the same thing. But improving your body isn't just about how you shop for food. That's just the beginning of my new 14-Day Plan, because when you get those groceries home you aren't going to believe what happens when you start cooking. The foods on my plan will naturally help you feel fantastic as you lose unwanted weight, and the recipes themselves will have you burning calories in ways you never imagined!

14 (FAT-BURNING) DAYS TO FABULOUS

My 14-Day Plan consists of three simple strategies that will change your life.

1. **Turn your kitchen into a gym:** *That's right—hit the kitchen, not the gym! In my plan, you cook more of your meals at home in order to gain control of the ingredients that go in your body—and you'll burn calories in the process. When you do it my way, you'll see that the act of cooking is a bona-fide calorie burner. For example, you'll burn 81 calories baking my Cinnamon Apple Rice Bran Muffins (page 102) for breakfast, 112 calories preparing my Ham and Tomato Panini with Spicy Mayo (page 124) for lunch, and 161 calories making my Spaghetti with Asparagus Pesto and Pecorino Romano (page 170) when dinnertime rolls around. And for dessert (yes, there is dessert on my plan—and snacks, too!), if you whip up my Chocolate Mousse (page 220), which is 121 calories a serving, you burn 135 calories[1] just preparing it—a calorie deficit! All of my recipes have built-in calorie burn, which is why you will lose weight while you cook.*

2. **Choose foods that burn fat naturally:** *Follow a diet centered on fat-burning choices— plant foods, natural foods, microbiotic foods, and allergen-free foods—and ease off indulging in too much meat, dairy, gluten, and other foods that are threatening your weight and your health. All the recipes here are deliciously free of gluten, lactose, and refined sugar, three substances that have been known to interfere with health and metabolism. I'll introduce you to the Super 5 Fat-Burn Selections, and you'll want to eat this way for life.*

3. **Avoid impure, fat-promoting foods:** *Purchase locally grown, preferably organic, additive-free foods because they're either low or devoid of hidden, stealthy substances called "obesogens" that are making you fat without your knowledge. I'll tell you more about obesogens, and how to avoid them, in Chapter Three, but most of all, I'll introduce you to a world of great-tasting healthy foods that you'll love. The best diets don't just tell you what you* can't *have and leave you stranded—they give you loads of great-tasting foods that you can eat without feeling guilty, which is what my plan does.*

These three key strategies are the cornerstone of my program, and each of the three chapters that follows explores every one in more detail, leading up to more than seventy-five recipes for breakfasts, lunches, dinners, snacks, and desserts, plus two full weeks of menus, that will help you lose eight to ten pounds in fourteen days. I'll also give you shopping lists, tips for stocking your pantry and fridge, information on where to find ingredients, and what brands I like best.

---

[1] This is my number based on my weight and fitness level; the actual number of calories burned depends on your weight and fitness level—your number could be even higher!—but there's no question that you will expend calories while you cook. See Chapter One for more on "cooking to burn."

Start your new adventure into cooking by following the recipes in this book. If you have basic kitchen skills, you can make these recipes—and you'll be delighted with your results, both on the table and on your body. By choosing the fat-burning food choices I offer here, your weight will start to melt off, practically automatically. And the health and vitality you'll enjoy from eating natural foods will convince you to change your nutrition and food-buying habits for good. I want you to love fresh and natural foods as much as I do and eat this way for life.

WHY 14 DAYS OF HEALTHY EATING CAN LEAD TO A LIFETIME OF GOOD HEALTH

After fourteen days on my plan, you will lose weight—eight to ten pounds, if you consume and burn the calories outlined on the program. Imagine how great you'll feel when you discover that the calorie burn on some recipes exceeds the amount of calories you consume when you enjoy the results! Guilt-free eating doesn't get any better or easier.

But it doesn't stop on Day 14. The three core nutritional strategies I'm introducing here can be followed for life, once you begin to explore all the foods available to you that fit the plan and learn to adapt your own recipes to this healthier way of cooking and eating. After fourteen days you'll experience noticeable results in how you look and how you feel. Your clothes will fit better. You may have to go shopping for a smaller size. Your energy levels will soar. Your skin will glow. All of this happens because you're nourishing your body with food that does not do damage to your system but in fact makes it stronger and healthier. At the end of fourteen days, you'll be telling yourself, "I love this way of eating," and you'll want to continue it indefinitely.

The right food choices and recipes are part of a healthy lifestyle, and I want to help you maintain your well-being for a lifetime—a long, happy lifetime. As we say in Italian, *"Salute!"*—to your health!

And as we say in English, get in the kitchen and *Cook Your Butt Off!*

PART ONE

THE PLAN

CHAPTER 1
Cook and Burn Calories

Strategy #1: Turn Your Kitchen into a Gym

SOMETIMES in life, there's a simple solution to a frustrating problem standing right in front of us. Literally.

Walk into your kitchen right now and go stand in front of your stove or your fridge or your pantry—and I promise that you're now standing right in front of the solution. The problem is how to burn more calories each day in order to lose weight or keep your weight under control. The solution lies in something that may surprise you: cooking at home, for yourself and for your family.

Sure, you already know that eating at home is generally less of a fattening affair than going out for double-bacon cheeseburgers, onion rings, and beers or a super-sized cherry cola. But it's not just what winds up on your plate—it's *how it gets there,* and that's what this first strategy is all about.

You may find this hard to believe, but *every hour you spend cooking and preparing food can burn up to 200 calories,* on average. If you're having a 400-calorie dinner—let's say my delicious Chili-rubbed Chicken with Black Bean Salsa and Rice (page 154), a piping hot Corn Muffin (page 210) on the side, and Mint Chocolate Chip Flurry (page 224) for dessert, you can burn half the calories from what you eat for dinner merely by cooking it yourself!

As a weight loss strategy, counting calories goes in and out of style, but there is no getting around the fact that controlling calorie intake and output is an important part of weight loss. Calories are a way to count how much energy is in food. Think of calories like gas. In the same way that gas makes your vehicle run, calories fuel your body. You use the energy you get from food to do the things you need to do daily: from breathing, thinking, cooking a meal, even sleeping, to bigger activities, like working out or running a race. However, when you don't expend the calories you've taken in (maybe you decide to skip your workout today), those calories get stored as fat, and you gain weight. To lose a pound, you have to burn about 3,500 calories.

So let's do a little arithmetic. Two hundred calories a day, 365 days a year is 73,000 calories. Divide that by the 3,500 calories that constitute each pound, and that 200-calorie difference will cause you to lose twenty-one pounds a year, automatically, when you prepare at least one meal a day and take an hour to do it. If you're ambitious enough to cook a second meal daily, double the numbers—you could be forty-two pounds lighter by the end of the year. So, without having to think about scheduling a structured exercise session, you can lose weight naturally just by getting in the kitchen and doing your thing.

Hit the gym? That can be a great way to burn calories, but it's so much easier to hit the kitchen, too—and get the same results!

COOKING AND CALORIES: PUTTING IT TO THE TEST

I regularly check the calorie-burn potential of cooking a meal by strapping a heart-rate monitor to my arm, one that calculates calorie expenditures (see below). Then I get to work and have fun watching the calories burn off. I didn't always wear a heart-rate monitor when I cooked (though I've been in the habit of using one for my triathlon training), but one day I decided to try it while I whipped up a simple meal for four. On the menu: vegetable lasagna, tossed salad, and fruit compote for dessert.

Heart-Rate Monitors 101: How to Buy a Great Heart-Rate Monitor

There are lots of heart-rate monitors out there. The best ones have the following features:

Bold display. *Make sure the screen is easy to read while you're working out, with large, clear numbers. Training at night? Make sure the screen has a backlight feature.*

User-friendly. *The monitor should be easy to set up, easy to use during your workout, and without complicated instructions.*

Accuracy. *Make sure the device is accurate, or it will do you no good. Have someone—preferably a qualified personal trainer—take your heart rate manually while you wear the monitor. Then compare readings.*

Alarms. *Use a monitor that has alarms to let you know when your heart rate leaves a zone.*

Stopwatch. *A stopwatch lets you time your exercise session.*

Continuous heart-rate reading. *Make sure your monitor can display a constant reading of your heart rate to determine if you're training at the right intensity.*

Virtual trainer. *I love this feature. It creates an exercise plan for you based on your training preferences and goals. The heart-rate monitor will give you the appropriate intensity and duration needed each day to achieve those goals.*

Uploading capability. *It's nice to be able to upload your training data from the monitor to your computer. That way, you can keep track of your progress.*

Comfort. *It's best if you can't feel or notice the monitor when it's strapped to your chest or wrist. I prefer monitors made of cloth rather than plastic because they're more comfortable.*

User-replaceable battery. *Get a monitor that allows you to replace the battery yourself without having to send the device back to the manufacturer when the battery runs out.*

I started the calorie-burn process by walking to my neighborhood market (and back) to buy the ingredients for the meal. They filled two shopping bags, which I carried home (always a great biceps workout!). After unloading the groceries, I checked the monitor out of curiosity. I had already incinerated about 158 calories. Walking (or biking) to and from the market is a great way to kick off your calorie-burning kitchen workout.

I sliced about a half-dozen squash and zucchini into long, flat strips, spritzed them with cooking spray, sprinkled them with salt, pepper, and thyme, and roasted them in a hot oven until crisp-tender. Meanwhile, I diced a bunch of tomatoes, chopped onions and garlic cloves, and sautéed them with Italian seasoning to make a marinara sauce. Finally, I blended some eggs and dairy-free cheeses by hand to create a spreadable filling.

When everything was ready, I layered a casserole dish with gluten-free lasagna noodles, strips of the roasted veggies, the marinara sauce, and the cheese filling. I poured the remaining sauce over the top, sprinkled with more shredded cheese, and baked the whole thing until warm and bubbling.

More chopping and dicing was in order to make a salad of romaine lettuce, sliced grape tomatoes, chopped green bell pepper, and Italian dressing that I shook vigorously before tossing with the salad. I peeled and sliced a few mangoes and some strawberries and layered them with sweetened soy yogurt in parfait glasses. Into the fridge they went to chill for dessert.

Calorie check: I had burned 228 calories slicing, roasting, dicing, sautéing, and moving quickly around the kitchen. After everyone had inhaled the meal that night, I began the process of kitchen cleanup, with the monitor still on my arm. Loading the dishwasher and scrubbing some of the more stubborn pots and pans burned an additional 106 calories. My grand total for the meal, from shopping to cooking to cleanup, was 492 calories. Considering that the meal was around 500 calories per serving, I had burned up nearly every calorie I ate that night.

After that experience, I can't even cook without wearing my heart-rate monitor because I might miss an opportunity to review my calorie expenditure or add to my weekly calorie burn. I do this, and yet I'm not training for my favorite physical activity—triathlons—or anything else. Consequently, I feel rewarded by the end of the week when my monitor gives me a summary of calories burned during cooking. This may sound like obsessive behavior, but it's fun and encouraging to know that I'm burning more calories making the stuff than I might be gaining by eating it. Take a look at the chart below to get an idea of how many calories you might expend in a single night of cooking.

FOOD PREPARATION ACTIVITIES	Calories Burned per Hour, by Weight			
	130 LBS	155 LBS	180 LBS	205 LBS
Baking	148	176	204	233
Bartending	136	162	188	214
Cooking or food preparation, including use of manual appliances (standing or sitting)	59	72	82	93
Cooking or food preparation (some walking)	89	106	123	140
Food shopping with or without a grocery cart (standing or walking)	77	92	102	121
Serving food, setting the table, clearing the table	89	106	123	140
Washing dishes (standing)	77	92	107	121
Washing dishes and clearing dishes from table (some walking)	89	106	123	140

Note: The numbers above are estimates. Individual calorie burn varies. The real number of calories burned in an activity varies with a person's size and fitness level, including body fat and muscle mass, as well as with the intensity of the activity. Source: Calculations are based on research data from Medicine and Science in Sports and Exercise, *the official journal of the American College of Sports Medicine; and data from www.calorielab.com.*

THE CALORIE BURN OF THESE RECIPES

As I got to work on the recipes in this book, I wore my heart-rate monitor. I wanted to see how many calories were burned when I prepared these recipes.

I was stunned. And what I discovered was certainly unexpected: Many of the calorie expenditures for these recipes were so high that they exceeded the calorie count of the actual recipe. For example, if you whip up my Banana Super Yogurt (page 114), which weighs in at 70 calories a serving, you burn 97 calories just preparing it! In other cases, you'll burn off a percentage of the calories in a dish when preparing it. Either way, you're burning, baby!

I'll say it again: Cook your butt off and burn calories—lots of calories!

Little Bites, Big Mistake: The High (Calorie) Cost of Nibbling

Yes, cooking can burn calories, but you just need to remember not to eat all the results of your dish. When I was a restaurant chef, I was always surrounded by food. To do my job well, I'd taste everything I cooked. Once I realized how many calories I was consuming by doing that, I stopped nibbling and started taking little tiny licks. And so should you, or it will cost you! Take a look:

Licking the spatula while baking cookies: **75 calories**

Pinching off a piece of roast beef when it comes out of the oven and popping it in your mouth: **68 calories**

Biting into a roasted Brussels sprout to test doneness: **15 calories**

Tasting a spoonful of mashed potatoes to check the seasoning: **42 calories**

Stuffing your mouth with a misshapen baked biscuit: **106 calories**

Sipping a glass of wine while cooking: **125 calories**

Damage: **431 calories—before you even sit down to eat!**

HOME IS WHERE THE BEST FOOD IN TOWN IS

Now you know that it's really possible to cook your butt off, but burning calories isn't the only reason to eat at home. When you prepare your own food in your own kitchen:

You eat better, you eat less (and you weigh less): People who dine out a lot, particularly at takeout joints or fast-food restaurants, are more likely to be overweight or obese than people who eat at home. When you prepare your own meals, the foods you make tend to have less salt, fat, and calories, not to mention mysterious ingredients and unwanted additives; home-cooked meals are just more nutritious than what you get at most restaurants. And although you *can* overeat at your own table, home-prepared portions tend to be smaller than the portions you get at restaurants. Research shows that we tend to eat what's in front of us, so if you polish off a burger and fries (a meal that totals about 1,000 calories), you've eaten about half the calories you should consume in the entire day.

It's good for you—and great for your family: Studies show that kids and teens who have three or more meals a week as a family are more likely to maintain normal weights and healthier diet habits than their peers who share fewer than three meals a week with their families. Bottom line is that you control portion sizes, and the content and quality you're serving your family. Once they've learned that good food is delicious *and* healthy, they're going to take that knowledge with them. I see this experience as a gift you're giving them that will last for the rest of their lives. I know this is true, because I inherited a love for good food from my own family. These issues really count in an era of rising childhood and adult obesity. Another benefit of eating at home as a family? Studies repeatedly show that kids who eat with their parents not only develop healthier eating habits, but also do better in school, are less likely to abuse drugs and alcohol, and share more information, communicating better with the caring adults in their lives.

You'll be thinner—and your wallet will be thicker: Boom! That's the sound of me blowing up one of the biggest food myths around: that cooking at home is expensive. Well, you may argue, "My favorite takeout joint is only thirty bucks for dinner for four—that's only $7.50 apiece." (Hmmm, do takeout three times a week, and you're spending nearly $100 a week.)

That same $30 could last you for three, maybe four meals if you cook at home. If you're averaging two takeout meals at those prices, that's more than $3,000 a year you're handing over in exchange for extra calories you and your family can do without. Why not stash that money away in a savings account to use on something more lasting than stuffed-crust pizza, like a vacation that you'll remember? If you have kids, they'll benefit more from a healthy college fund than they will from an unhealthy order of chili-cheese fries! I'm not going to tell you how to spend your money, but I will tell you that many people are under the misconception that shopping for good ingredients and preparing great food is expensive. Yes, you can spend a lot of money on imported balsamic vinegar, or heirloom tomatoes, but those are specialty items or are used sparingly; the everyday staples that are part of a healthy kitchen don't cost a fortune.

Want to know what I do to save money and calories? Here are some tips, and all of these suggestions work perfectly with the recipes and meal plans in *Cook Your Butt Off!*

I eat more meatless meals like my Chili "Cheeseburger" that uses meaty-tasting portabello mushrooms, for example, and I snack on fruit instead of highly processed snack bars. I don't use high-priced convenience foods, either. And I prefer to cook with gluten-free grains and choose fruits and vegetables that are in season—always a cheaper deal. When I'm thirsty, I drink water, not juice or soda. It's cheap—free, if I drink filtered tap water, and free of the added sugars found in soda and the extra calories in juice. Or I drink my own refreshers such as my Apple, Lime, and Basil Smash (page 76) and my Prickly Pear Chamomile Cooler (page 78).

Also, I like to buy in bulk. A can of black beans might cost about $1.50, but the equivalent amount of organic dried black beans in bulk is around 40 cents or less. I buy items like beans, nuts, grains, and spices in bulk and save money; plus, I always have great quality staples on hand when I want them. Bulk foods don't use much packaging, either, a bonus for environmental protection. I like to spend Sunday afternoons cooking big batches of soup, sauces, or casseroles, and then freeze the food in portion-sized containers for later use.

I love shopping at farmers' markets and buying locally grown, responsibly raised foods—as you'll see in Chapter Three, it's also a great smart and economical way to stock your kitchen.

One of the best ways to save $50 to $100 a month is to go to the grocery store with a list and buy only what's on the list. When you buy extra items, that's where overspending comes in and how you can go over your budget.

Use coupons and shop for discounts. Shop weekly store specials for your meat, dairy, and produce, and bring along coupons for your favorite healthy foods. (But watch out—many big food manufacturers love to offer deep discount coupons on junky new processed foods to lure buyers. Don't take the bait!) Take a look at the store's weekly circular and target the best deals for your menu planning, plus check out couponing sites like www.retailmenot.com.

Finally, the real cost of not making your own food goes beyond cash and calories. We've been living too long under the delusion that mass-produced food, cheaply made with sugars, fats, and nasty additives and preservatives, is acceptable. It's just the opposite: It's a health horror story. The escalating rates of heart disease, diabetes, cancer, and other diet-related diseases prove it. Put another way: You think kale is expensive? Try heart disease and type 2 diabetes.

I know that if you're really hooked on eating out, then cooking your meals at home is going to take some added effort, and you'll need to ease into it. It does take discipline, but it also yields life-changing results—and remember the calorie burn! It really makes a difference.

COOK TO LIVE, LIVE TO COOK

The next two strategies will focus on foods to eat and foods to avoid, but both steps assume that you'll be ready and willing to get into the kitchen and prepare your own meals based on those foods. Cooking for yourself is key to making this plan work, and I hope I've given you enough reasons as to why it's totally worth it.

My goal has always been to get people to cook and to discover the rewards and pleasures of the kitchen. When you cook healthy, great-tasting meals for yourself, you're treating your body with the respect it deserves. When you cook with the same care and enthusiasm for others, you're sending a message that their happiness and well-being matters to you. Every time you cook a meal, you're reconfirming your devotion to those you are feeding.

I call this cooking with love. It's something you can't taste, but it's something you can feel. It doesn't matter if it's a humble bowl of soup or an elegant five-course meal; if food is cooked with love, you will never forget it. It is the most important ingredient when you cook for people you care about. When you cook, whether it's breakfast just for you or dinner for your whole family, cook your butt off—with love.

ROCCO'S RULES FOR TURNING YOUR KITCHEN INTO A GYM

Still think you need to go to a pricey, crowded spin class to burn calories? From shopping to prep to cleanup, here are some tips for heating up your calorie burn (without blowing bucks on a gym membership):

- *Park your car as far as you can from the grocery store entrance. Better yet, don't drive to the market—walk or bike there!*

- *Walk briskly around the store as you shop. If you aren't buying a lot of items, carry a small basket with you instead of pushing a cart. You'll move more quickly and you'll work your arms as you fill your basket.*

- *Avoid pre-cut produce. Buy whole vegetables and fruits—and peel, chop, dice, or slice them yourself. They'll be fresher (and cheaper) if you DIY.*

- *Go low tech and high energy for maximum calorie burn. Skip the food processor and put some energy into your knifework. (Added bonus: Your knife skills get better with practice.) Forget the stand mixer and blend, beat, and whisk with good old-fashioned elbow grease. Put some muscle into it!*

- *Stay on your feet during food prep; it burns more calories than sitting on a stool or chair. Even if you're not actively moving from stove to counter to fridge, just standing burns more calories than sitting. Sore hips or knees? Feeling tired? Treat yourself to a kitchen "gel mat," and standing (and burning calories) becomes a lot easier.*

- *Pick up the pace while moving around your kitchen. Crank up your radio and dance around the kitchen as you prepare your food and clean up later.*

- *Burn more calories during kitchen cleanup: Wash pots and pans yourself instead of plopping down in front of the TV while your partner or an electric dishwasher does the job.*

- *Sweep and mop the kitchen floor, scrub down the sink, and polish up the stovetop. All these things burn calories (and your kitchen will be nice and clean!).*

- *Take a long walk or bike ride after dinner for one last blast of calorie burning.*

- *And don't forget to wear a good heart-rate and calorie-counting monitor when you cook!*

CHAPTER 2
Eat and Burn Fat

Strategy #2: Choose Foods that Burn Fat Naturally

WHEN you want to lose weight, calories count, but so do your food choices. The foods you choose matter—because some foods can cause you to pack on fat, while others help you burn it right off. When you modify your calories *and* choose the right foods, you mount a two-pronged attack against fat that results in faster, easier weight loss.

The recipes and diet plan in this book are based on choosing the fat-burners and steering clear of the fat-makers:

THE SUPER 5 FAT-BURN SELECTIONS

When you eat foods from these five categories, you'll watch your weight melt off and your overall health soar. I call these groupings the **Super 5 Fat-Burn Selections**. These foods are on my list of kitchen must-haves, and I cook with them regularly. The latest science shows that foods in the Super 5 contribute to healthy weight loss, and they help to fight certain chronic illnesses. You will feel great and look great when you cook and eat the Super 5 way!

1. NATURALLY SUGAR-FREE FOODS

Sugar will screw with your weight and your health. It was the first "calorie hog" to go from my diet years ago. Little by little, I reduced my overall sugar intake, including my sweetened beverage consumption, a huge source of liquid sugar (and calories) we don't always keep track of. Most

11

beverages, from sodas to flavored coffees—even the ubiquitous energy drink—are just not worth the weight-damaging sugar and calories (see below). I still treated myself to dry wines on occasion, though, since they contain virtually no sugar. The change in my health and energy levels was revelatory, and the difference I felt in my system was incredible.

BIG GULPS OF SUGAR (BY BEVERAGE CATEGORY)			
BEVERAGE	SERVING SIZE	CALORIES (RANGE)	TEASPOONS OF SUGAR (RANGE)
Fast-food Smoothie	1 medium	310 to 602 calories	15 to 34 teaspoons
Frappuccino	16 ounces	230 to 400 calories	12 to 15 teaspoons
Bottled Teas	16 ounces	180 to 220 calories	11½ to 13½ teaspoons
Bottled Flavored Milk	13 to 16 ounces	300 to 340 calories	11½ to 13½ teaspoons
Sodas	12 ounces	143 to 170 calories	9½ to 12 teaspoons
Energy Drinks	8 to 8.5 ounces	110 to 140 calories	7 to 8 teaspoons
Juice and Fruit Drinks	8 ounces	70 to 160 calories	4½ to 9 teaspoons
Vitamin Waters	12 ounces	75 calories	5 teaspoons

SUGAR CONTENT IN ALCOHOL—THE BEST AND THE WORST			
BEVERAGE	SERVING SIZE	CALORIES (RANGE)	TEASPOONS OF SUGAR (RANGE)
THE BEST (LOWEST IN SUGAR CONTENT)			
Beer	12 ounces	55 to 153 calories	0 teaspoons
Distilled Liquor (bourbon, gin, rum, Scotch, vodka)	1½ ounces	96 to 103 calories	0 teaspoons
Wine, red, dry	1 medium glass (5.1 fluid ounces)	117 to 127 calories	¼ teaspoon
Wine, white, dry	1 medium glass (5.1 fluid ounces)	114 to 122 calories	¼ teaspoon
THE WORST (HIGHEST IN SUGAR CONTENT)			
Piña Colada	8 fluid ounces	437 calories	14 teaspoons
Long Island Iced Tea	10 fluid ounces	300 calories	10 teaspoons
Mojito	10 fluid ounces	428 calories	10 teaspoons

Tequila Sunrise	10 fluid ounces	348 calories	7 to 8 teaspoons
Wine, red or white, sweet	1 medium glass (5.1 fluid ounces)	230 calories	5 to 8½ teaspoons
Liqueurs	1 shot (1.5 fluid ounces)	112 to 159 calories	2 to 6 teaspoons
Margarita	10 fluid ounces	464 calories	4 to 5 teaspoons
Cosmopolitan	4 fluid ounces	213 calories	3 teaspoons

When I refer to "sugar" in our foods, I'm talking about refined (not naturally occurring) sugars that are dumped into foods and beverages, such as high-fructose corn syrup, sucrose, or any sugar with a chemical name that ends in "-ose." Not long ago, the American Heart Association issued a document on Dietary Sugars Intake and Cardiovascular Health. It concluded that Americans are on a sugar binge, and that's the major reason why more than one-third of us are overweight. On average, we're consuming 22 to 30 teaspoons of sugar a day. That's 350 to 475 lethally sweet calories that boost the risk of disease.

The problem with sugar is that, simply, it jacks up the hormone insulin. And when your insulin levels go up and stay up, you pack on fat. Eventually, your pancreas (which manufactures insulin) will start wearing down, and then you're staring at type 2 diabetes.

The best way to eat sugar free is to choose foods in their most natural state so that you can get the full benefit of their nutrients. When you stick to natural foods, such as fruits, veggies, certain grains, and lean proteins, your diet is automatically low in sugar. Stay away from most packaged foods (which are typically loaded with sugar) and sugar-sweetened beverages like sodas and "juice drinks" (which are usually sugar water with barely any real juice).

Hey, I love sweets as much as the next person. After all, I'm a chef, so living in New York City and traveling all over the world only developed my love for all things scrumptious and sugary. But I know sugar calories are empty, nasty calories. So I've done a lot of experimenting to come up with some great-tasting recipes that will satisfy your sweet tooth without refined sugar. They harness the sweetening power of the following ingredients, which you'll see in my recipes (you'll also find information in the recipes on brand names and instructions on how to use these sweeteners in their various forms).

Monk Fruit

Let me introduce you to the newest sweetener on the block: monk fruit, a small green melon that has been grown in Asia for centuries. Supposedly, it got its name from Buddhist monks who cultivated the fruit in southern China. The fruit provided folk remedies for common ailments like colds and constipation. Today, the fruit is crushed, mixed with hot water, filtered, and spray-dried to form a sweet, zero-calorie powder, now used in a number of foods and beverages, from granola to cocktails. Monk fruit is 300 times sweeter than sugar, and you can cook with it.

Does it have any negative side effects? Not that anyone can tell. People in Asia have enjoyed monk fruit for eons, with no observed negative health outcomes. In May 2012, the prestigious Academy of Nutrition and Dietetics published a position paper on low-calorie sweeteners supporting the safety of monk fruit sweeteners.

Palm Sugar

Resembling brown sugar, palm sugar (also called coconut sugar) comes from the sap of palm trees. It contains tiny amounts of minerals including calcium, iron, magnesium, phosphorus, potassium; the B vitamins riboflavin and thiamin; as well as trace amounts of protein. Unlike white sugar, it helps reduce the speed of the blood sugar rush. Palm sugar also contains beneficial antioxidants, according to a February 2010 study in *Food Chemistry*. You can typically find this healthier sugar in Southeast Asian, Indian, or Central American markets, or grocery stores that stock a good selection of natural foods.

Mixing palm sugar with stevia, a non-caloric sweetener, cuts the calories, plus intensifies both sweeteners.

Coconut Nectar

This sweetener is made from the sweet juice that drips off coconut flower buds. It, too, contains nutrients not found in refined sugars: seventeen amino acids, as well as a bunch of minerals and vitamins B and C.

Granulated coconut nectar has a caramel/maple flavor and can be used in place of brown sugar in recipes. I love it on top of fruit or toast, in hot cereals, and for baking.

Erythritol

This is a no-calorie sweetener I occasionally use in recipes. It occurs naturally in fruits such as grapes, pears, and watermelon, as well as in foods like wine and cheese. Erythritol is technically a sugar alcohol, but don't worry, it won't get you drunk. Nor is it as taxing on the digestive system as other sugar alcohols. It performs well in baking.

Stevia

I've used stevia in its powdered and liquid forms for a long time, and with good results. This sweetener is extracted from the eponymous South American herb and is estimated to be as much as 400 times sweeter than sugar. It has no calories and can be used safely by people with diabetes without hiking up blood sugar or otherwise influencing glucose levels. To bake with it, use 1½ tablespoons powdered (or 1 teaspoon liquid) stevia for 1 cup sugar. It takes some experimentation to achieve the right sweetness.

Grown-Up Uses for Baby Food

I'm cooing over cooking with baby food. It's an excellent fat substitute and natural sweetener. It helps seal in moisture in baked goods, too. There's no fat, salt, or added sugar in it, either—one of the purest and most natural foods you can get. If you're whipping up a fruit or vegetable bread, use two (7½ ounces each) jars of baby food carrots, pears, and mashed bananas to liven things up. I use baby food prunes in my Asian Pork Buns (page 162) as part of the sauce; it's amazing. Get creative with baby food. You can't go wrong.

Where's the Fat?

Not on my 14-Day Plan, that's for sure. I use very little fat when I cook these days. I prefer to rely mostly on olive oil cooking spray, so stock up on it. I am absolutely enamored with this product. It's my go-to condiment when preparing low-fat dishes. Normally, you'd use it to keep food from sticking. But it has even more ingenious uses to create "you'd-never-believe-it's-low-fat" foods. Spray it on a crumb coating for a fried-food taste in fish or chicken. Spray it on lettuce for a virtually no-fat Italian-like dressing. Spray it on veggies or other foods to crisp them up while baking. Spray it in your skillet to sauté meats and veggies. I've found that the uses are practically endless—which is why it is the predominant "fat" I'm using for food preparation in these recipes. A one-second spray contains less than a gram of fat, compared to nearly 14 grams of fat (and about 120 calories) in 1 tablespoon of oil—and they do virtually the same amount of work.

2. DAIRY ALTERNATIVES

If you've given up dairy products, you're a member of a growing club, and I'm in it. Many people are cutting out dairy for a variety of reasons: They might be sensitive or intolerant to lactose (naturally occurring sugar) or the proteins (such as casein) found in dairy products. They want to reduce animal fats and cholesterol in their diets. Or they want to avoid indirect exposure to the synthetic hormones and antibiotics injected into dairy cows to boost milk production.

But here's the scary part: Apart from encouraging weight gain, some dairy products contain a hormone called IGF-1 (insulin-like growth factor 1), which may make cancer cells proliferate. Our bodies already make IGF-1 naturally, so when we eat dairy products that contain IGF-1, we might be overdosing on a hormone that triggers cells in our bodies to multiply abnormally. Furthermore, there is some evidence that the milk protein casein may be a carcinogen. Studies published by Cornell University have shown a link between the casein in the food of lab mice and liver cancer. The jury is still out as to whether casein promotes liver cancer in people, but for some of us, the lab studies are enough to make us think twice about consuming cow's milk.

Foods High in Lactose and Casein

The most common high-lactose and high-casein foods include:

- Milk, milkshakes, and other milk-based beverages
- Whipping (heavy) cream
- Ice cream, ice milk, sherbet
- Certain cheeses
- Butter
- Puddings
- Cream soups, cream sauces
- Foods made with milk

Source: www.clevelandclinic.com

A big question I am frequently asked about a dairy-free diet is, "How do I get enough calcium?" Sure, our bodies require this essential mineral to maintain strong bones, govern hormones, and make sure our muscles (including the heart, which is a muscle) and nerves work properly. The good news is that certain green leafy vegetables and legumes (such as spinach and black-eyed peas, for starters) supply all the calcium you get from cow's milk and other dairy foods but without the animal fat and the potential health risks.

Most chefs don't like to eliminate items from their recipes, but when I decided to take charge of my health and eat less dairy, I spent a lot of time devising recipes to replace dairy in cooking. I now use a lot of nut milks, soy milks, and dairy-free cheeses, and you can't tell the difference.

Some of my recipes call for dairy cheese, though, but it's optional. The two dairy cheeses I prefer are Parmigiano-Reggiano and Pecorino Romano. Parmigiano-Reggiano is a 100 percent lactose-free cheese. Its name comes from the Parma and Reggio Emilia regions in Italy, where it is produced (it is also produced in Modena and parts of Bologna and Mantua). The cheese is made with skimmed cow's milk and processed to the highest standards. Italian mountain climbers pack chunks of this cheese instead of energy bars for quick energy, since the body can absorb the protein from Parmigiano-Reggiano in forty-five minutes, faster than it can soak up the protein from other cheeses.

Pecorino Romano is low in lactose. That means if you're lactose sensitive, you can probably enjoy it. This type of cheese is a sheep's-milk cheese. To know you're getting the real thing, look for the outline of a sheep's head on the label or look for established brands such as Locatelli. Pecorino Romano is a grating cheese like Parmigiano-Reggiano, but it has a completely different taste. Also, Pecorino Romano should not generally be used instead of Parmigiano-Reggiano.

Other dairy foods you can enjoy if you're lactose sensitive include kefir and low-fat yogurt, both made from fermented milk and full of beneficial bacteria that is kind to your digestive system. Historically, kefir has been fermented from the milk from sheep, goats, and cows, but you can now buy soy milk kefirs. Kefir is drinkable. As for low-fat yogurt, it usually doesn't trigger lactose intolerance because the good bacteria in it help digest lactose. Soy yogurts are available, too, and they're even better than regular yogurt for lactose-sensitive tummies.

I don't necessarily advocate a dairy-free diet for everyone, but if you choose to lay off dairy there are more nondairy options available than ever before. The chart below gives a rundown on my favorite dairy alternatives—and why they do your body so much good.

MILKY WAYS

DAIRY ALTERNATIVE	HOW IT'S MADE	HEALTH BENEFITS	CALORIES PER 8 FLUID OUNCES
Almond Milk (unsweetened)	Made from a blend of nuts and water	Cholesterol-free, fat-free, lactose-free. High in vitamin E. Fortified versions supply additional vitamins and minerals. In a 2011 study published in *Nutrition and Cancer*, cow's milk stimulated the growth of prostate cancer in lab dishes; almond milk suppressed cell growth.	60
Coconut Milk (unsweetened)	Made from the grated meat of fresh coconut	Generous in minerals, especially iron. Contains a special type of fat that assists weight loss and weight maintenance.	50
Hemp Milk (unsweetened)	Made from a blend of hemp seeds and water	Allergen-free; high in protein, omega-3 fatty acids, vitamins, and calcium.	100
Rice Milk (unsweetened)	Made from a blend of rice and water	Cholesterol-free, fat-free, lactose-free, allergen-free.	120
Soy Milks, Yogurt, and Cheeses (unsweetened)	Made from cooked, ground soybeans and water	Low in saturated fat and abundant in magnesium, riboflavin, selenium, and omega-3 fatty acids. Soy milk is also lactose-free.	80

3. GLUTEN-FREE FOODS

More and more, I've been serving up gluten-free dishes—everything from chocolate cupcakes to chicken noodle soup to spaghetti—in response to the many folks out there who are making the decision to go gluten-free.

Some do it because they've received a medical diagnosis of celiac disease, a serious autoimmune disorder triggered by the protein gluten, which is found in wheat, barley, and rye. When someone with celiac disease consumes foods containing gluten, an autoimmune reaction is triggered that damages the villi in the small intestine over time. The damaged villi do not absorb nutrients from food, thus, the body is basically starved of the nutrition required to support life.

Other people stop consuming gluten—cutting out bread and bread products, baked goods, pasta, breakfast cereals, crackers, pretzels, and all other gluten-containing grain products—because they have a non-celiac-disease sensitivity to this protein, and they feel loads better when they remove it from their diets. (Note: Gluten is found primarily in products made from grains, but it also lurks in foods made with additives, like store-bought chicken stock and salad dressings.)

Gluten—which many consider toxic to the body—triggers chronic inflammation throughout the body if you're sensitive or allergic to it. That's pretty nasty stuff, since inflammation is linked to life-threatening illnesses such as heart disease, cancer, stroke, Alzheimer's disease, diabetes, kidney disease, osteoporosis, inflammatory bowel disease, and rheumatoid arthritis. A study in the *New England Journal of Medicine* listed fifty-five health problems eating gluten can trigger or worsen.

Many people are going gluten-free to control their weight—a connection scientists are just beginning to study. Researchers at the Universidade Federal de Minas Gerais in Brazil recently published an interesting study examining the metabolic effects of gluten. They rounded up some lab mice wanting to drop a few sizes and put them on a gluten-free diet. After eight weeks, the mice lost fat tissue, decreased inflammation, and handled insulin better. Lab animals are one thing, but will a gluten-free diet work for humans? Scientists say yes—for a couple of reasons:

- ***Gluten instigates the production of substances called exorphins that can have addictive effects on your body.*** *Like addictive drugs, exorphins trigger a desire in your brain that makes you crave gluten-containing foods, which, in turn, could contribute to weight gain, since gluten is found mostly in high-carb foods. A craving for carbs could actually be a craving for gluten.*

- ***Gluten triggers leptin resistance, which causes overeating.*** *The hormone leptin sends signals to the brain that you're full and don't want any more food. In other words, leptin keeps your hunger in check so you don't overeat. That's how things work if you're healthy* *and at your ideal weight. It's different for overweight and obese people. They have what scientists have termed "leptin resistance," in which cells rebel against leptin and do not register the correct hunger signals. Grains, especially the gluten-containing ones, are thought to promote leptin resistance and therefore weight gain and obesity, according to a study by researchers published in the December 2005 issue of* BMC Endocrine Disorders.

- ***Most commercially produced gluten-containing foods are processed, and often loaded with refined sugar, so you're getting lots of extra and empty calories that might get stored as fat.*** *When you decide to avoid gluten, you're naturally eliminating the kinds of foods that contribute to weight gain and make it hard to permanently keep the weight off—foods like chips, doughnuts, pretzels, cookies, muffins, bagels, pasta, pizza, sugary cereals, beer, most commercial French fries, and more.*

The fact is that the optimum diet for weight loss should be either gluten-free or at least lower in gluten. I'm going to make this easy for you, because you'll find mostly gluten-free foods on my 14-Day Plan. Some recipes do have gluten, but in these cases, I'll give you substitutions. What's more, my recipes introduce you to a whole new world of gluten-free foods and replacements. See the chart below for foods that are safe to eat and foods that contain gluten. The section that follows introduces you to some of my favorite ingredient substitutes, items that you'll see in the recipes in Part 2 of this book.

Here's the bottom line: Regular bread and I have had a long relationship, so I know what it's like to break up. If you're a bread lover (as I was), you may find the idea of saying good-bye to gluten hard to handle, but trust me: Whether you're motivated to give up this potential toxin because it triggers so many unpleasant effects in your system, or whether you're looking for the game-changer that will help you lose weight once and for all, you will not regret removing it from your diet. And these days, you can find all sorts of delicious gluten-free breads and other baked goods, so breaking up isn't as hard to do. The best diets aren't just about removing foods. They're about replacing certain foods with healthy alternatives, which is the goal here. And you don't have to go cold turkey. Remove gluten gradually if you decide to give it the heave-ho. That's the easiest strategy.

NATURALLY GLUTEN-FREE FOODS	HIGH-GLUTEN FOODS
Beans, seeds, nuts in their natural, unprocessed form	Barley (malt, malt flavoring, and malt vinegar are usually made from barley)
Fresh eggs	Rye
Fresh meats, fish, and poultry (not breaded, batter-coated, or marinated)	Triticale (a cross between wheat and rye)
	Wheat

NATURALLY GLUTEN-FREE FOODS

Fruits and vegetables

Most dairy products

Certain grains: amaranth, arrowroot, buckwheat, corn and cornmeal, flax

Gluten-free flours (rice, soy, corn, potato, bean)

Hominy (corn)

Millet

Quinoa

Rice

Soy

Tapioca

Teff

Gluten-free pastas: brown rice pasta, corn pasta, quinoa pasta, shirataki noodles, soy pasta

HIGH-GLUTEN FOODS

Bulgur

Durum flour

Farina

Graham flour

Kamut

Semolina

Spelt

GLUTEN-CONTAINING PRODUCTS

Avoid these unless labeled "gluten-free" or made with corn, rice, soy, or other gluten-free grain:

Beer

Breads

Cakes and pies

Candies

Cereals

Cookies and crackers

Croutons

French fries

Gravies

Imitation meat or seafood

Matzo crackers and meal

Pastas

Processed luncheon meats

Salad dressings

Sauces, including soy sauce

Seasoned rice mixes

Seasoned snack foods, such as potato and tortilla chips

Self-basting poultry

Soups and soup bases

Vegetables in sauce

Source: www.mayoclinic.com

A FEW OF MY FAVORITE THINGS

When you're getting rid of gluten, sugar, and other calorie hogs, you've got to hunt for creative substitutions. The following ingredients are the newest finds in my healthy, low-calorie cooking repertoire. Stock up on them! You'll want to have them on hand once you start cooking from my 14-Day Plan.

INGREDIENT	BENEFITS	USES
Arrowroot	A fine white powder valued for its thickening ability and neutral flavor. Another advantage is arrowroot doesn't cause a sauce or gel to become cloudy or opaque.	Dissolve arrowroot in a cold liquid before whisking into a hot liquid. This mixture is called a "slurry," and you'll use it as the basis for certain sauces, stocks, and gravies. Look for arrowroot powder in the spice section of the supermarket.
Egg white powder	Made from dried egg whites, this ingredient is very healthy, with none of the fat or cholesterol you find in eggs. The powder is an easy way to lower the calories in recipes.	This powder makes a great binder for pancakes, latkes, and meat loaf—any mixture in which the ingredients require adhesion. You can also reconstitute the powder with water to make scrambled eggs, meringues, and other items requiring egg whites. Look for egg white powder where supplies for cake baking and decorating are found.
Pectin	A fiber found in many fruits.	Pectin is used as a thickener and in jams and jellies. Like fat, pectin helps to keep baked goods tender (which is why high-pectin products like applesauce and fruit butters can replace a certain amount of fat in baked food recipes). You can find it in the baking section of your supermarket.
Psyllium husks	A grain, high in fiber, used in some bulk-forming natural laxatives and in some breakfast cereals. It helps slow down the release of sugars. There is strong evidence that this fiber curbs hunger to help with weight loss and prevent weight gain and obesity.	Use the ground husks as a low-carb, low-glycemic grain to replace all or some of the flour in recipes. You'll find psyllium husks in health food stores and whole-foods markets.
Puffed brown rice	A form of rice cereal created by forcing steam inside the hull. The rice is then pressure cooked or baked or fried, causing the grain to swell and expand. Puffed brown rice is high in vitamins, minerals, and fiber.	Use the cereal as a bulking agent in foods such as meat loaf or crushed as a coating for fish and poultry. Puffed rice cereal has a much better nutrition profile than basic bread crumbs, which are normally used in these types of recipes. You'll find puffed brown rice in the cereal aisle in most grocery stores.
Rice bran	This is the brown layer removed when the white rice kernel is processed. Rice bran reduces unhealthy cholesterol levels as effectively as oat bran does, according to studies.	Use it in desserts to replace all or some of the flour. It has a natural sweetness that curbs the amounts of sugar needed in recipes. You'll find rice bran in health food stores and grocery stores that stock a good selection of natural foods.
Shirataki rice	A rice-like product made with yam flour (konnyaku), with no fat, gluten, or preservatives, and practically no calories.	It is best used in soups and stir-fry. The main source for this product is online at www.miraclenoodle.com and whole-foods markets.
Soy pasta	An alternative starch that is high in protein and gluten-free.	Use this pasta as a replacement for traditional wheat pastas. It is available at most grocery stores.
Xanthan gum	A strong, versatile ingredient that can instantly thicken just about anything. It has a pleasant mouthfeel that will be perceived as fatty, although no fat is there.	On gluten-free diets, use xanthan gum in baking to replace the gluten. It is available in most gluten-free sections of grocery stores.

4. ALKALINE FOODS

Try to eat mainly alkaline foods. I'm a recent convert to eating this way, and it wasn't hard to make the leap. As an Italian through and through, I grew up on a Mediterranean-type diet, which is composed mostly of foods that are alkaline (think tomatoes, eggplant, red wine, and olive oil), with proportionally less meat and other acidifying foods.

An alkaline diet is basically about achieving the right dietary balance between alkaline and acidic foods, and creating a healthy blood pH level. You may eat both types of foods, but try to eat more alkaline foods than acidic ones. When your blood is more alkaline, you may lose weight more rapidly. One reason is that alkalinity zaps food cravings. It just follows that if your cravings decrease, you'll eat less.

Another reason is that this type of diet helps preserve muscle mass, and the more muscle you have, the more calories you burn. Alkaline foods like fruits and veggies are rich in potassium and magnesium, minerals that reduce acid load in your body, and help preserve muscle, according to a three-year study published in 2013 in *Osteoporosis International*.

On the other hand, acidic foods do, as the name suggests, create acids in the body. They can cause weight gain, bloating, fatigue, and other health problems. By contrast, alkaline foods help you control your weight, increase your energy, and promote overall well-being.

So, could your diet be too acidic? Signs include weight gain, poor digestion, bloating, fatigue, and dry or spotty skin. If so, it may be time to give alkaline eating a try.

Alkaline foods include fruits, vegetables, fruit juices, potatoes, and beverages such as red and white wine, green tea, and soda water. Grain products, meat, fish, dairy products, and pale beers tend to be more acidic. Here's a chart that explains which foods are alkaline and which are acidic.

	TOP ALKALINE FOODS	TOP ACIDIC FOODS
DAIRY	Acidophilus milk	Cheddar (reduced fat)
	Buttermilk	Cottage cheese
	Whole milk	Hard cheese
	Yogurt	Parmesan cheese
		Processed cheese
EGGS	Egg whites	Egg yolks

	TOP ALKALINE FOODS	TOP ACIDIC FOODS
VEGETABLES	Basil Broccoli Cabbage Carrots Celery Cucumber Eggplant Garlic Green beans Lettuce, all varieties Mint Onions Parsley Parsnips Pumpkin Soybeans Spinach Sprouts Squash Tomato Turnips Water chestnuts Watercress Most vegetables, with the exception of those in the acid column	Asparagus tips Garbanzos Lentils
PROTEINS	Tempeh Tofu Whey protein powder	Cod Corned beef Frankfurters Lean beef Luncheon meat Trout Turkey Veal
FATS AND NUTS	Almonds Butter Chestnuts (roasted) Coconut (fresh) Flaxseed Margarine Olive oil Vegetable oil	Peanuts Walnuts

	TOP ALKALINE FOODS	TOP ACIDIC FOODS
GRAINS AND GRAIN PRODUCTS	Amaranth Millet Quinoa	Cornflakes Rice, brown Rice, white Rolled oats Spaghetti, regular Spaghetti, whole grain
FRUITS	Apples or apple juice, unsweetened Apricots Banana Blackberries Black currants Blueberries Cherries Grape juice, unsweetened Grapes Lemon Lime Melon, all varieties Orange juice, unsweetened Oranges Passion fruit Peaches Pears Pineapple Plums Raisins Raspberries Tangerines Watermelon Most fruits with the exception of those in the acid column	All preserves Any fruit canned with sugar Cranberries Olives (pickled) Prunes
BEVERAGES	Beer, draft Coffee Green tea Wine, red Wine, white	Alcoholic beverages

Adapted from: Schwalfenberg, G. K. 2013. The alkaline diet: is there evidence that an alkaline pH diet benefits health? Journal of Environmental and Public Health 2012:1-7.

I recommend that three-quarters of what you eat be alkaline and the rest be acidic to help place your body into the right balance. My 14-Day Plan is primarily alkaline and will help you get started on this way of eating.

5. MICROBIOTIC FOODS

When you eat a meal, there are trillions of microbes in your stomach that are eating, too. Known as gut microbiota, these bacteria help control our weight and are directly connected to obesity. They extract calories from what we eat, help store those calories for later use, and yield energy and nutrients for the production of new, helpful bacteria to continue this work. They also affect our appetite and, possibly, even what foods we crave.

The research into microbiota and obesity took off in 2006, when scientists at Washington University in St. Louis noticed something unusual: Fat mice and skinny mice have very different bacteria in their guts. Could different bacteria actually cause obesity, they wondered?

To find out, the scientists took gut bacteria called firmicutes from obese mice and put them into thin ones. The thin mice ate their normal diet—no more, no less. Nonetheless, they quickly started putting on pounds (or should I say, ounces). Firmicutes, it turns out, are really good at packing calories away as fat, much better than the common gut bugs called bacteroidetes. This may be why your best friend can wolf down fattening food and stay skinny, while you gain weight from merely looking at cheesecake. It seems that if you have fewer firmicutes and more bacteroidetes, you can burn off many more of, say, the 400 calories in a hot fudge sundae. Scientists now suspect that overweight and obese folks have too many firmicutes in their gastrointestinal tract.

Gut bacteria, in the right balance, can be beneficial, even vital, when it comes to maintaining good health. They may help prevent asthma, cardiovascular problems, and possibly even mood disorders. They protect against acid reflux, and they churn out many of the same feel-good chemicals as our own brains do. And they're great for digestion; you'll be surprised how easy it is to get your poop train running on schedule if your gut is well populated with good microbiota.

There are plenty of foods you can eat to achieve the optimum balance of microbiota in your system. One is soy yogurt, which I mentioned above and which I cook with a lot. It is made from soy milk and also contains live yogurt cultures and often, fruit. Soy yogurt is a great choice if you're lactose intolerant and/or want to remove lactose from your diet. So is kefir, another great microbiotic choice.

Other sources of microbiota include:

- ***"Stinky" vegetables.*** *Onions and garlic, for example, are rich in the prebiotic fiber inulin. Prebiotics are foods that feed good bacteria in the gut and help them multiply. Other stinky foods include cabbage and Brussels sprouts, both good sources of prebiotics.*

- ***Chewy foods.*** *Chewiness can indicate fiber, too, which is why (gluten-free) steel-cut oats, quinoa, and brown rice are more nutritious to the microbiota than more processed grains.*

Beware of diets too high in protein and low in carbs and fiber. These diets are associated with a microbiotic profile linked to colon cancer. And here's where refined sugar and saturated (animal) fats rear their ugly heads: Diets laced with refined sugar and saturated fats may stimulate the growth of toxic bacteria in the gut—bacteria that can turn against us and make us sick. You'll find that my plan and recipes are loaded with foods that help beneficial microbiota survive and thrive.

ROCCO'S RULES FOR CHOOSING FOODS THAT BURN FAT NATURALLY

Strategy #3, coming up next, will help you figure out what foods to avoid. But Strategy #2 is all about what foods to eat and which ingredients to choose when you cook your butt off. So remember:

- ***Eat from the Super 5 Fat-Burn Selections.*** *There are fantastic options for replacing sugar, dairy, and gluten in your diet. Eat from my plan and stick with the Super 5!*

- ***Up the alkaline on your plate.*** *You can still eat acidic foods, but make sure most of your foods are alkaline, for better health and weight loss.*

- ***Do a gut check.*** *Pay attention to the millions of miraculous microbiota in your gut. When they're in balance—through a healthy diet—you're going to find that weight loss and good health come easily!*

CHAPTER 3
Cook Fresh, Stay Lean

Strategy #3: Avoid Impure, Fat-Promoting Foods

I EAT natural, organic, and local foods most of the time, and I'm very conscious of the ingredients in the foods I eat. I like to know what goes in my food. I'm a big label reader, and I don't like the look of anything that lists additives I can't pronounce. I do this because many of our foods contain substances that are not necessary for life or good health. Many of these substances include artificial fats, refined sugars, pesticides, additives, and unnatural hormones, and they present real threats to our health. Even though this stuff appears in tiny amounts in food, its impact on our well-being can be huge, causing problems such as heart disease, cancer, allergies, and obesity. Here is what you should steer clear of:

FATTENING CHEMICALS: MEET THE OBESOGENS

Among the most notorious fat triggers are chemical substances known as obesogens. Obesogens are technically defined as chemicals—both manmade and naturally occurring—that make you fat. Obesogens can be added to foods as ingredients, such as high-fructose corn syrup and MSG, or they can wind up in our food supply during its production; for example, hormones given to animals that wind up in our food chain, and the pesticides that are sprayed on our food.

Obesogens make us fat, and they do this subtly, but in different ways. For one thing, they mess with the body's normal metabolism and its hunger hormones. Their worst offenses are to screw with the release of leptin (which keeps us from overeating); to encourage the body to store fat; to reprogram cells to become fat cells; and to encourage insulin resistance (which leads to diabetes).

For more than a decade now, scientists have been scratching their heads over why there has been such a surge of obesity worldwide. People are cutting calories, fats, and carbs—even exercising more. Yet we're still getting fatter. Now those scientists have turned their attention to obesogens for an explanation, and research into the issue has been heating up. Biology professor and researcher Bruce Blumberg, who first coined the term *obesogens*, was quoted in the journal *Environmental Health Perspectives* in 2012 as saying: "I would not want to say that obesogen exposure takes away free will or dooms you to be fat. However, it will change your metabolic set points for gaining weight. If you have more fat cells and propensity to make more fat cells, and if you eat the typical high-carbohydrate, high-fat diet we eat, you probably will get fat."

So in addition to burning more calories and choosing more fat-burning foods, you've got to avoid obesogens. It's not quite as simple as reading labels (though that helps tremendously—bye-bye, high-fructose corn syrup!), but if you're aware of where obesogens lurk, you can avoid them.

The main places you'll find these scary fat-making chemicals are:

MEAT

It's no secret that U.S. farmers raise millions of cattle to be turned into juicy steaks, prime rib, sumptuous roasts, and hamburgers. What you may not know, however, is that a majority of those cattle are fattened up with hormones—hormones that are similar to steroids taken by bodybuilders and athletes. Other cattle are given female hormones like estrogen. In male cattle, this synthetic estrogen chemically castrates the animal (ouch!), enabling them to grow faster. In female cattle, estrogen shuts down the menstrual cycle, thereby devoting more of the cow's energy to fattening up. (Estrogen is a fat-forming hormone.)

Besides the hormones that we wind up ingesting when we eat our steaks and burgers, a substantial portion of these hormones literally passes through the cattle into their waste and ends up in the soil, where it can get into our food and drinking water. These foreign hormones have been implicated in some studies as one of the causes of the drastic rise in obesity. When we consume hormone-injected meat or foods grown in hormone-contaminated soil, those chemical substances go into our bodies, changing our metabolism so that we store more fat.

Of course, this is all very bad news for me. I love beef. I've been a sworn carnivore since birth. I would be happy if, after I'm old and wrinkly, I got hired to do those "Where's the beef?" commercials. I won't let anyone take away my beef, but, if you're like me, there are actions you can take to reduce your exposure to these kinds of obesogens:

- *Buy the leanest cuts of meat you can, since hormones get stored in the fat of beef.*

- *Purchase only organic, grass-fed and/or pasture-raised meat, poultry, and eggs.*

- *Choose only cuts labeled "no antibiotics added" or "certified organic."*

- *Ease off your intake of meat, perhaps to only one serving a week. Why not compromise and eat just half the amount of animal protein you ate before? Doing so also decreases your risk of heart disease and cancer, anyway.*

- *Experiment with more meatless recipes, such as the ones you'll learn here.*

DAIRY

What I just mentioned above in regard to meat goes for dairy, too. Many dairy farmers pump their animals with hormones to increase milk yield—and these hormones could be linked to the obesity epidemic.

To avoid obesogens in dairy, one solution is to go dairy free, or at least milk free. Some suggestions:

- *Develop a taste for nondairy milks, made from nuts, like almond milk or coconut milk; from grains, like rice milk; or from vegetables, like hemp or soy milk. (See pages 15—17 in Chapter Two for lots of ideas on dairy alternatives.)*

- *Try dairy-free versions of sour cream, cheese, and ice cream.*

- *Pump up your calcium intake from leafy greens, sardines, beans, shrimp, crab, and calcium-fortified nondairy milks.*

- *Still love dairy? Try to cut back on your overall consumption of dairy products, and use only organic products.*

PESTICIDES

Pesticides and fungicides sprayed on produce, or found in farm-raised fish, act like estrogen in the body and disrupt natural thyroid hormones, which regulate metabolism. The net effect is that these obesogens, like hormones, encourage weight gain.

The best ways to avoid this danger:

- ***Buy certified organic foods.*** *They haven't been sprayed or treated with pesticides, fungicides, or other chemicals.*

- *If you can't find or afford all-organic produce, take a look at the charts below from the Environmental Working Group.* *If you do purchase conventional (as opposed to organic) produce, at least you can safely choose the "clean" fruits and veggies with confidence.*

- *Purchase fish raised in environmentally healthy environments,* *or known to be wild-caught, fished, or farmed in healthy ways. See the chart below for examples of the best seafood choices in the categories:*

BEST WILD-CAUGHT FISH	BEST WILD-CAUGHT SHELLFISH	BEST FACTORY-FARMED FISH	BEST FACTORY-FARMED SHELLFISH
Cod	Blue crab	Cobia	Clams
Halibut	Clams	Pompano	Crawfish
Mackerel	Lobster from Mexico and New England	Bass from Spain	Oysters
Mahimahi			Scallops
Perch	Oysters		Shrimp
Pollock	Scallops		
Salmon	Snow crab		
Sea bass			
Swordfish			
Tuna, albacore and yellowfin			

Note: A complete resource here is www.seafoodwatch.org. The organization publishes an extensive chart on the best and worst seafood choices.

- *Note that almonds, peanuts, and pecans are likely to be heavily sprayed, so always buy organic versions of these nuts; pesticide residue can make it through their shells.*

- *Wash your fruits and veggies thoroughly under running lukewarm water and peel off outer layers of leafy vegetables. Using lemon juice or baking soda helps remove residue, too, as does using a vegetable scrub brush on harder-surface fruits and vegetables.*

Fruits and Veggies with the Highest Levels of Pesticide Residue—The Dirty Dozen™

1. Apples
2. Celery
3. Cherry tomatoes
4. Cucumbers
5. Grapes
6. Hot peppers
7. Nectarines—imported
8. Peaches
9. Potatoes
10. Spinach
11. Strawberries
12. Sweet bell peppers

Fruits and Veggies with the Lowest Levels of Pesticide Residue—The Clean Fifteen™

1. Asparagus
2. Avocado
3. Cabbage
4. Cantaloupe
5. Sweet potatoes
6. Eggplant
7. Grapefruit
8. Kiwi
9. Mango
10. Mushrooms
11. Onions
12. Papaya
13. Pineapple
14. Sweet peas
15. Cauliflower

Source: Environmental Working Group, www.ewg.com

HIGH-FRUCTOSE CORN SYRUP (HFCS)

This chemically derived version of corn syrup is a big-time obesogen. It's found in most processed foods, including commercially baked bread, sodas, crackers, and cookies. The body metabolizes HFCS differently from refined sugar, converting it straight into fat. This conversion process may also raise levels of triglycerides (fat in the blood), which are implicated heavily in heart disease. Eliminating HFCS from your diet may help you lose excess weight and improve your overall health.

Here's my advice on how to start:

- **Avoid packaged breads, crackers, and other snacks containing HFCS** *(you'll want to do this anyway if you're eliminating gluten and refined sugar from your diet).*

- **Break the fast-food habit.** *Fast foods often contain HFCS, even if they don't taste sweet.*

- **Eliminate soda from your diet.** *It's little more than HFCS and carbonated water.*

- **Read labels of foods to make sure they do not contain high-fructose corn syrup, corn syrup, or fructose.** *It's in places where you might not expect it, such as canned soups and spaghetti sauce.*

Label Reading 101

When I was a kid, I put the cereal box in front of me on the kitchen table while I was eating my breakfast. I would read the label on the box as I spooned the cereal into my mouth. I loved this ritual. I didn't understand everything on the label; nonetheless, it was fascinating.

Today, I read labels for health reasons, since they're packed with data that can help me make better choices. If you're new to label reading, here's a crash course on the key parts of the label with which to be most familiar.

- Serving size. Check this part first. Many packaged foods and beverages contain more than one serving. For example, in a 1-cup bag of trail mix, the serving size is ¼ cup, so one pouch contains 4 servings.

- Calories. If you're losing or controlling your weight, keep your eye on how many calories are in the particular food—per serving size. Too many calories can turn into too much body fat, although the quality of your calories matters, too.

- Dietary fiber. We need to be eating 20 to 35 grams of fiber a day. Knowing the amount of fiber in foods helps get you to this goal, so this number is very important to check.

- Total fat. This is the tally of all the types of fat found in the food, including saturated, trans, monounsaturated, and polyunsaturated. Choose products with fewer grams of total fat per serving.

- **Saturated fat.** This is artery-clogging fat in beef, pork, poultry, full-fat dairy products, and butter. Limit your saturated fat to 7 percent or less of your daily calories. That means 15 grams or less for most of us.

- **Trans fat.** This nasty fat is worse than saturated fat; limit intake to less than 2 grams per day, if any. If the words "partially hydrogenated" appear on the ingredient list, the product contains trans fat. (Trans fat is being phased out of all foods, fortunately.)

- **Cholesterol.** Here's a good number to check if you have heart health concerns. If you have heart disease, limit cholesterol intake to 200 milligrams (mg) or less per day, and 300 mg or less for others.

- **Sugars.** Keep an eye on this number. One teaspoon of sugar equals 4 grams, so if the nutrition label lists the sugars content at 16 grams, it's equivalent to 4 teaspoons of sugar. Sugar—whether in the form of honey, corn syrup, molasses, glucose, fructose, or cane sugar—will jack up your blood glucose level fast. This can lead to health problems, even narrowed arteries.

- **Ingredient list.** Scan this list before you toss a food into your grocery cart. If you see that highly refined ingredients, such as white flour, white rice, and sugar, appear high up on the list, the product is probably a very processed food. Look for chemicals, too, such as additives, colorings, and preservatives—usually items you can't pronounce or don't recognize. The addition of chemicals also indicates the food is highly processed and probably unhealthy.

REPLACING BAD FOOD WITH GOOD FOOD: THE LOCAL SOLUTION

I shop at farmers' markets, food co-ops, and whole-foods-type stores, so I regularly see the amazing abundance of fresh, healthy, and delicious food our country is capable of producing. That's why it drives me nuts to see the stuff that dominates our diets and takes up most of the real estate in a typical grocery store—a mess of industrialized, globalized foods that are disconnected to any factor of good health.

Too much of our food is laced with bad fats, refined sugars, artificial flavorings, chemical additives, pesticide residues, obesogens, genetically modified organisms (GMOs), and other harmful things that do not belong in our bodies. Too much of it is grown without a thought to how its production may be damaging our environment for future generations. But there are ways to fight back, beginning with what foods we choose to bring into our kitchens and put on our plates.

FROM FARM TO TABLE

I've become increasingly conscious of how our food is produced, and where—and who—it comes from. I've always preached that fresh is best in terms of overall food quality and nutrition. But—and this is a big "but"—the produce you buy in your grocery store may not be truly fresh.

Scallions that are harvested in Mexico, transported by truck or plane to the States, and sent cross-country to your local supermarket are still labeled fresh (as in, never frozen), even though they were picked from the patch days or weeks ago. Apples from the West Coast might be picked and kept in cold storage for a year before being shipped to the East Coast. It's been documented that most food travels an average of 1,500 miles before landing on our plate.

So what does that do to our fruits and veggies?

For one thing, produce may lose some of its nutrient value when it's transported over long distances. A tomato, for example, is picked before it's ripe so it travels better (rock-hard refrigerated tomatoes won't bruise as easily as ripe ones, but they sure won't taste as good). When the tomato is picked too early, it is considerably lower in nutrient value than a tomato grown slowly and allowed to naturally ripen on a small non-factory farm.

As for animal products, you just read about the hormones and antibiotics that we ingest when we eat factory-farm raised meats, and don't even get me started on how animals are raised in those settings. Chickens are often so pumped up with hormones to increase the amount of breast meat that they can barely move.

For these reasons, it's a good idea to purchase meat, poultry, and eggs locally, too—particularly from non-factory farms, where you can usually get organic, pasture-raised, and free-range foods. Livestock that lived and grazed on grass yield meat, poultry, eggs, and dairy products that are more nutritious than the same foods from grain-fed animals, especially those raised in confinement. Case in point: An Argentine study published in the journal *Meat Science* in 2005 revealed that grass-fed meat is higher in vitamin C, vitamin E, and beta-carotene than its grain-fed counterpart.

What's more, meat from pasture-fed chickens, ducks, geese, and turkeys is leaner than that from factory-farmed poultry, and that meat is more nutritious. Eggs from pastured chickens have darker yolks, harder shells, and more nutrients than eggs laid at factory farms.

Meats, poultry, and eggs that have been raised responsibly and naturally will be labeled as such, so look for labels such as *grass-fed, organic, pasture-raised,* and *free-range* when you buy these foods.

I'm definitely a big advocate of supporting local farms, farmers' markets, and roadside stands, where you have direct access to a wider and much fresher variety of fruits and vegetables, as well as healthier meat, poultry, and eggs, than those available at the grocery store. You are buying locally, which also means you are helping the environment by buying products that haven't been shipped thousands of miles. And best of all, the products are the freshest they can be with all the flavor and nutrients they should have.

Get to know your farmers, too—where they grow their products and how they're grown, as well as how they raise their livestock. Farmers can answer questions, suggest how to prepare and cook their product, and offer information about the food. Can you get that from the cashier or stock person at the supermarket?

10 Reasons to Cook Your Butt Off with Locally Grown Foods

1. **Flavor.** *Fruits and vegetables that have been picked within a day or two taste better, because they've been able to ripen in the field—no long-distance transportation, no gassing to stimulate the ripening process, no sitting for weeks in storage.*

2. **Seasonality.** *The food you buy at the farmers' market is seasonal and meant to be ripe at a certain time of the year. That's when it tastes best, too. This is also another great way to boost your overall health.*

3. **Humane treatment of animals.** *At the farmers' market, you can buy meats, cheeses, and eggs from animals that have been raised humanely, without hormones or antibiotics. These animals have grazed on green grass and been fed natural diets. And they've been spared the overcrowded living conditions found at big corporate factory farms.*

4. **Environmental protection.** *Factory farms use methods that pollute the water, land, and air, whereas small farms grow foods using methods that minimize the negative effect on the earth.*

5. **Nourishment.** *Food purchased at farmers' markets is minimally processed and nutrient dense, since farmers work hard at building the soil's nutrient content. Those nutrients are passed on to us when we eat the food.*

6. **Variety.** *You'll find a wider variety of produce at a farmers' market than you'll see at conventional grocery stores.*

7. **Income for your local growers.** *Buy locally, and you help farmers keep their land. You are supporting individual people and the local economy, not massive agribusiness that genetically modifies food. Plus, you're keeping money circulating in your community. This in turn benefits other businesses.*

8 . **Safety.** *Food from your local farmers is generally safer. Remember those scary outbreaks of E. coli from bagged spinach? These things occur mostly as a result of handling and processing in large food conglomerates, where quality control can sometimes lapse.*

9 . **Meet your farmer.** *You and your kids can actually talk to the farmers, learn about their methods, and then decide for yourself before you buy. In most cases they will let you come and visit their farms.*

10 . **Family fun.** *Shopping at a farmers' market is a social experience for your whole family and one that allows you to connect with your community. There are often activities for kids and other vendors selling crafts. I would much rather stroll amid outdoor stalls of fresh produce on a sunny day than push my cart around a grocery store with artificial lights, frigid air conditioning, and piped-in music.*

I know what you're thinking: Isn't it more expensive to shop and eat like this?

Not really—and yes, I'm going to address the cost issue again. Locally grown food is generally cheaper because it's in season and it's not traveling halfway across the world. When foods are out of season, prices are dramatically higher because they are being imported from far-flung places. If you want sticker shock, buy asparagus in December. The asparagus season is in the spring and lasts only about six weeks. If you realize this too late, you'll miss out on buying it at its cheapest, which is around $2 a pound. Out of season, it jumps to more than $3 a pound.

Before you head to the supermarket, map out your menu for the week. This will help cut your trips to the grocery, as well as impulse buys. Buy vegetables, herbs, and salad greens au naturel—rather than washed, cut, and stuffed in sealed bags—because they're less costly that way. They also won't be contaminated with anything foreign, other than a bit of dirt from the fields. I'll never forget the time I stuck my hand in a bag of lettuce and got stung by a wasp. That was the last time I ever bought bagged lettuce.

As for organic meats, I won't lie to you: They are a little more expensive. Just eat less of them, since a plant-centered diet will always be healthier. When you think about what goes into factory-farm-raised animal products, you'll reach for the organic ones. They are so much better for you that the price really is worth it.

Garden Programs

Another way to save, if you've got the time, is to grow a few of your own vegetables. You can grow most vegetables in large containers placed on a balcony or deck. In the early fall, plant vegetables such as spinach, lettuce, broccoli, cabbage, turnips, and radishes, and herbs such as parsley, chives, and garlic. As summer gets close, plant summer veggies like tomatoes, peppers, and cucumbers.

I've found that growing my own vegetables offers a harvest of benefits. They taste better and are fresher than anything I can buy. I know for sure that they're pesticide free. I love stepping out on my balcony and picking fresh produce for dinner. And I love enjoying the fruits of my labor.

If you don't have the time to grow veggies, consider joining a Community Supported Agriculture (CSA) organization. These groups link small farms to individuals. You buy a "share" from a farmer. The share is typically a box or basket of vegetables, sent to you at certain times during each farming season. For information on how to subscribe to a CSA, check out the website www.localharvest.org/csa.

ROCCO'S RULES FOR AVOIDING IMPURE, FAT-PROMOTING FOODS

- *Steer clear of obesogens, and get educated on where they're hiding.* They pop up in meats, dairy, produce, and fish.

- *Toss out anything in your kitchen with high-fructose corn syrup.* This is a real baddie when it comes to obesogens. You don't need it, and you won't miss it.

- *Go local, not global.* You don't need food from halfway around the world if a farmer is selling it at your local greenmarket. Buy in season, and when you can, choose organic produce and meats.

Cook your butt off with good ingredients and real food from nature. Next up: The plan you've been waiting for, complete with recipes and menus.

CHAPTER 4
Cook Your Butt Off in 14 Days

ARE you ready? Because here it comes—my 14-Day Plan for cooking your butt off, including recipes and four weeks' worth of menus. You know the three strategies now:

Strategy #1: **Turn your kitchen into a gym.** (Burn calories while you cook.)

Strategy #2: **Choose foods that burn fat naturally.** (Remember the Super 5!)

Strategy #3: **Avoid impure, fat-promoting foods.** (Go natural, get thin.)

You can eat

- *Delicious, easy-to-prepare recipes, with nutrient-packed ingredients*
- *Two fresh fruits daily, preferably organic and locally grown*
- *Microbiotic foods, alkaline foods, and other plant-based foods, all in a healthy daily balance*
- *Two daily snacks (recipes included)*

You don't have to worry about

- *Counting calories. I've already counted them for you; simply follow the menu plans, and you'll automatically be cutting calories to a level at which pounds will peel off. That level is 1,200 calories a day.*

- *Feeling hungry. The 14-Day Plan is loaded with foods and beverages that will keep you full and satisfied.*

- *Allergic reactions. I can't say it too many times or in too many ways: This plan frees you from potential allergens because it has no gluten, lactose, and refined sugar. Because of this, you won't experience any bloating, digestive irritability, skin problems, fatigue, or other factors associated with food reactions.*

You'll limit (or cut out, depending on your preferences)

- *Red meat*

- *Cow's milk and other dairy products*

- *Wheat products and gluten-containing foods*

- *Refined foods such as white rice and white flour*

- *Refined sugar*

- *Too many acidic foods*

It might look like you're cutting out a lot of foods—but not really. You're actually adding in more foods that you may be eliminating. Take a look:

LIMIT/AVOID	SUBSTITUTE
Butter, margarines	Olive oil, olive oil cooking spray, avocados
Meats	Organic, grass-fed meats; lean meats; reduced serving sizes; plant proteins such as beans and legumes; soy derivatives (tofu, soy yogurt, soy cheeses)
Milk	Almond milk, coconut milk, hemp milk, rice milk, soy milk
Dairy	Dairy-free foods (such as soy cheese, soy yogurt, tofu)
Eggs	Egg white powder, egg whites; egg replacements (such as Egg Beaters); tofu
Some factory-farmed fish	Wild-caught fish and responsibly farmed fish
Refined cereals	Any acceptable gluten-free, sugar-free cereal, such as puffed brown rice

Refined sugars	Monk fruit, palm sugar, coconut nectar, stevia
Sodas and diet sodas	Fresh water, coffee, green tea, herbal tea, any of the many beverage recipes in this book
Wheat pastas	Soy pastas, shirataki noodles
Wheat and gluten-containing foods	Amaranth, arrowroot, brown rice, buckwheat, corn and cornmeal, flax, hominy (corn), millet, quinoa, rice, soy, tapioca, teff
White rice	Brown rice, puffed brown rice, shirataki rice
White flour	Gluten-free flours (rice, soy, corn, potato, bean)

WHEN YOU DON'T HAVE TIME TO COOK: READY-MADE SUBSTITUTIONS

Hey, I'm a realist. I know you don't always have time to cook. And I know you're not clamoring to spend a whole lot of time in the kitchen. To help you out here, I'll be giving you suggestions for healthy, low-calorie, low-fat meals that you can just pop in the microwave or oven. These products are basically prepackaged meals, along the lines of TV dinners. Swap a recipe out for one of these products, and you've got yourself a great substitution that will help you shed pounds. They're generally balanced and contain a mix of protein, carbohydrate, and fat, as well as other nutrients.

Using these meals saves time and takes the guesswork out of meal planning. They're also a great option if you prefer to eat foods that are already calorie and portion controlled for you. And they're useful if you struggle to control or understand portion sizes.

At the end of most of my recipes, you'll see my suggestion for a ready-made substitution that can stand in for that particular recipe.

Cook Your Butt Off with These Special Tools

This book is not about fancy sauces, glossy emulsions, or changing the texture of foods for the sake of gastronomy. Rather, it is about you and your health, not about what fancy (and expensive) equipment you park in your pantry. Although I'm not asking you to buy a new fleet of kitchenwares, I would like you to get a few items that will make your food prep a little easier:

- **Digital Scale.** Measure everything! Measure everything! Measure everything! Unless you have the visual eyesight of an eagle you will never be able to guess. So control calories from the start and measure all your ingredients. A decent digital scale that measures to the tenth of a gram is less than $20.

- **Sturdy cutting board.** Chopping is a great calorie burner. For best results, use a large-surface, flat, heavy-duty cutting board. Smaller cutting boards put you more at risk for injury. At home, I use one that is 20 inches long and 12 inches wide (it is actually a carving board that I use during the holidays but turned upside down so that the juice channel is not in the way).

- **Sturdy box grater.** Have on hand a good old-fashioned grater with four sides of varying grating surfaces.

- **Microplane rasp grater/zester.** This tool is a handheld, super-sharp grater. My favorite is the Microplane Classic Zester, available wherever kitchen tools are sold.

- **Mason jars.** Sometimes called "Ball jars" (Ball being a popular brand), these are reusable glass jars that have tight-fitting lids and are designed for canning and preserving. I like them because you can not only mix or shake in them, but also serve beverages in them. Unlike most plastic smoothie bottles, they are made of glass and thus environmentally friendly.

- **Meat mallet.** This item is a heavy tool that comes in a variety of shapes and sizes. I prefer one with both a flat and a textured side. Although mallets are widely available, you can use a flat-bottomed, heavy-duty pot or pan with a sturdy handle to do the work of the mallet.

- **Mortar and pestle.** Here's a great invention that dates back to ancient Egyptian medical practices. It has so many uses, from making powders of spice, coffee, or dehydrated fruits and vegetables to making great pastes of fresh herbs and citrus zests. If you don't want to buy one, you can simply chop very finely with a heavy-duty chef's knife and use the side of the chef's knife to smash the foods.

SUGGESTED MENUS FOR THE 14-DAY PLAN

It's going to be easier than you think to get in the groove of this new way of eating. To help you get started, I've created fourteen days of menus for you. If you're someone who doesn't like to make decisions about meals and what to eat, simply follow the plan verbatim—there's no guesswork involved when you take this route.

On the other hand, if you like to do your own thing, or if you find that you love certain recipes and want to repeat them, you can substitute those for the meals I've listed. The recipes are organized into Beverages, Breakfasts, Lunches, Dinners, Salads and Soups, Snacks, and Desserts. Simply slot in what you want to eat for each meal from my recipes.

I've done my best to create menus comprised of foods and recipes that have broad appeal, but if you cannot eat or simply don't want to eat what I have proposed, then simply swap it out with something similar. For example, where you might see an apple for a snack, and you don't want an apple that day, simply substitute it for another fresh fruit of roughly the same weight and calories (use those produce scales in the supermarket!).

You can pick and choose among the recipes and arrange them anyway you like. You will lose weight rapidly on this plan—and start feeling fantastic right away. Plus, most experts agree that it takes only fourteen days to lose your taste and desire for sugar, gluten, and fat. In a matter of days, this way of eating will be your "new normal" and definitely not a default diet. Also, each recipe makes a single portion, but you can easily double, triple, or quadruple it for extra servings. Each day's menu nets you around 1,200 calories, an amount designed to take weight off steadily, especially if you're exercising—and cooking your butt off!

About dining out: If you want to go out, I don't recommend you do so more than a few times a week, max. This plan is most effective if you follow it closely. Going out or getting takeout for dinner several nights a week will definitely set you back. You want to take advantage of the calorie burn of cooking these dishes and making this way of eating second nature.

MY EXPERIENCE

Remember that the 14-Day Plan is more than just a two-week diet; it is a whole new blueprint for healthy eating. At the end of fourteen days, expect to feel lighter, more energetic, and younger looking. Check in with yourself and see how you feel at the end of two weeks. That's exactly what I did. Call it self-experimentation with me as the guinea pig. I gave myself two weeks to stay off sugar, gluten, and lactose. After doing that, my workouts improved; I had more energy to do more. My gastrointestinal system got more tuned up (that is all I will say—you can fill in the blanks!). Mentally, I had more clarity and creativity. My skin improved. On and off throughout my life, I had been troubled with back pain, the result of standing on my feet all day and night in restaurants. I gave this stuff up for just two weeks, and the pain was gone. My life changed because I got rid of foods bad for my body, and gave it foods it demanded. It was a striking shift.

So—after your two weeks, do an inventory of how you feel, look, and perform after laying off these substances. I believe that the positive effects of this diet will inspire you to continue it for another two weeks—and beyond. What's more, expect your friends and family to ask you what you've been doing to look so good and be so energetic. Share this diet with them. Doing so might just motivate them to commit to this lifestyle change, too.

At the very least, I hope these benefits will inspire you to continue this way of living. To that end, be sure to read Chapter Five, Day 15 and Beyond, in which I give you realistic strategies for extending the plan beyond just two weeks.

Enjoy! (Recipes and instructions for preparation begin on page 73.)

DAY 1

		Cals	Fat G.	Carbs G.
BREAKFAST	Cocoa Crispies (p. 96)	97.5	2.3	19.5
	Strawberries, fresh, ½ cup halves	49	0.5	11.7
	Coffee or green tea	0	0	0
SNACK ONE	Apple, Lime, and Basil Smash (p. 76)	37	0	10
	Turkey Jerky (p. 214)	45	0	1
LUNCH	Wrap with Shrimp and Tomato Salad (p. 122)	177	6	13
	Add 1 tablespoon extra virgin olive oil	120	14	0
	Apple, small (6 ounces purchase weight)	80	0.3	21
	Water	0	0	0
SNACK TWO	Autumn Snack Clusters (p. 206)	114	0.5	25
	Walnuts, 1 ounce shelled	175	16.7	2.8
DINNER	Asian Pork Buns (p. 162)	182	4	26.75
	½ avocado	114	10.5	5.9
	Kimchi, raw, 7 tablespoons	25	0	5
	Coconut Clusters (p. 226)	91	5	13.85
	Water	0	0	0
TOTALS		1306.5	59.8	155.5

DAY 2

		Cals	Fat G.	Carbs G.
BREAKFAST	Greek Scramble with Tomatoes and Mint (p. 98)	78.3	1.6	5
	Turkey bacon	35	1.4	0
	Coffee or green tea	0	0	0
SNACK ONE	Chocolate Milk (p. 80)	40.5	2.3	5.75
	Banana, medium	105	0.4	27
LUNCH	Ham and Tomato Panini with Spicy Mayo (p. 124)	215.5	7.25	26
	Apple, medium (7 ounces purchase weight)	93	0.3	24.7
	Water	0	0	0
SNACK TWO	Grilled Sweet Potatoes with Spicy Coconut Nectar (p. 216)	147	4	23
	Hummus, 3 tablespoons, with ½ cup carrot sticks	75	3.1	10.8
DINNER	Chicken and Mushrooms Balsamico (p. 144)	152	3	14.075
	Heart of Palm and Escarole Salad (p. 188)	123	6	16.34
	Chocolate Mousse (p. 220)	121	7	15.25
	Water	0	0	0
TOTALS		1331.8	40.35	190.915

DAY 3

		Cals	Fat G.	Carbs G.
BREAKFAST	Living in Green Smoothie (p. 88)	109.25	0.25	21.25
	Hard-boiled egg, large	78	5.3	0.6
	Coffee or green tea	0	0	0
SNACK ONE	Turkey Jerky (p. 214)	45	0	1
	Fresh Fruit Salad	73.5	0.2	19.3
LUNCH	BLT Salad (p. 180)	140	6	14
	Turkey breast, store-bought, roasted on premises, 3 ounces	115	0.6	0
	Walnuts, ½ ounce shelled	88	8.4	1.4
	Water	0	0	0
SNACK TWO	Autumn Snack Clusters (p. 206)	114	0.4	24.8
	Banana	105	0.4	27
DINNER	Meat Loaf with Mashed Sweet Potatoes (p. 158)	175.5	3.4	10.6
	Corn Muffin (p. 210)	50	0.5	10
	Ice Cream Sandwich (p. 228)	95	5.25	13.5
	Water	0	0	0
TOTALS		1188.25	30.7	143.45

DAY 4

		Cals	Fat G.	Carbs G.
BREAKFAST	Sausage and Egg Breakfast (p. 104)	121	0.75	6
	Cinnamon Apple Rice Bran Muffin (p. 102)	65	1.85	11
	Coffee or green tea	0	0	0
SNACK ONE	Living in Green Smoothie (p. 88)	109.25	0.25	21.25
	Pumpkin seeds, dry-roasted, 3 tablespoons	120	11	4
LUNCH	Turkey and Avocado Sandwich (p. 126)	279	9	29
	Cherry tomatoes, 1 cup	27	0.3	5.8
	Water	0	0	0
SNACK TWO	Crispy Brown Rice Snack (p. 208)	95	0.5	22.75
	Banana, medium	105	0.4	27
DINNER	Spaghetti with Asparagus Pesto (p. 170)	208.5	5.5	35
	New Year's Resolution Sangria (p. 92)	28.5	0	9
	Sweet Potato and Chocolate Truffle (p. 230)	59	5	8.25
	Water	0	0	0
TOTALS		1217.25	34.55	179.05

DAY 5

		Cals	Fat G.	Carbs G.
BREAKFAST	Smoked Salmon and Yogurt Breakfast (p. 106)	128	2.7	12
	Grapefruit, ½ large	53	0.2	13.4
	Coffee or green tea	0	0	0
SNACK ONE	Pumpkin Pie Smoothie (p. 90)	59	1.5	11.7
	Stevia-sweetened dark chocolate, ¼ bar (10g)	80	7.5	11
LUNCH	Lentil Salad with Sherry Vinegar and Mirepoix (p. 192)	114	0.5	16.8
	Lean Pork Loin, store-bought, roasted on premises, 3 ounces	122	3	0
	Fruit Punch (p. 84)	7	0	2
SNACK TWO	Autumn Snack Cluster (p. 206)	114	0.5	24.8
	Water	0	0	0
DINNER	Cod with Tomatoes, Zucchini, and Olives (p. 156)	143	2.25	8.7
	Roasted sweet potato (3.9 ounces)	100	0.2	23
	Add 1 tablespoon extra virgin olive oil	120	14	0
	No-Bake Apple Pie Squares (p. 232)	94	0	22.25
	Water	0	0	0
TOTALS		1134	32.35	145.65

DAY 6

		Cals	Fat G.	Carbs G.
BREAKFAST	Pancakes with Coconut Nectar (p. 108)	89	0.3	18
	Grapefruit, ½ large	53	0.2	13.4
	Coffee or green tea	0	0	0
SNACK ONE	Iced Cappuccino (p. 82)	5	0.3	16.25
	Cinnamon Apple Rice Bran Muffin (p. 102)	65	1.8	11
	Add 1 tablespoon virgin coconut oil	120	14	0
LUNCH	Vegetarian Chili Burger (p. 128)	80	0.5	15.55
	Ketchup	10	0	4
	Lettuce	4	0	0.8
	Avocado	114	10.5	5.9
	Pink Lemonade (p. 86)	13	0	4
SNACK TWO	Turkey Jerky (p. 214)	45	0	1
	Banana	105	0.4	27
	Water	0	0	0
DINNER	Sweet Potato Spaetzle (p. 174)	205	0.2	37
	Cauliflower and Kale Salad (p. 190)	43	0.4	9
	Shrimp, steamed, 4 ounces	112	1.2	0
	Carrot Cake (p. 234)	90	1	9.5
	Water	0	0	0
TOTALS		1153	30.8	172.4

DAY 7

BREAKFAST		Cals	Fat G.	Carbs G.
BREAKFAST	Italian Zucchini Scramble with Tomatoes and Basil (p. 100)	66	0.5	8.5
	Grapefruit, ½ large	53	0.2	13.4
	Canadian bacon, 2 slices	87	4	0.6
	Coffee or green tea	0	0	0
SNACK ONE	Apple, Lime, and Basil Smash (p. 76)	37	0	10
	Cinnamon Apple Rice Bran Muffin (p. 120)	65	1.8	11
	Add 1 tablespoon virgin coconut oil	120	14	0
LUNCH	Crispy Tacos (p. 130)	172.5	2	31.75
	Turkey breast, skinless, store-roasted, 4 ounces	153	0.8	0
	Pink Lemonade (p. 86)	13	0	4
SNACK TWO	Crispy Brown Rice Snack (p. 208)	95	0.5	22.75
	Water	0	0	0
DINNER	Roasted Pork with Sauerkraut and Apples (p. 164)	220	4.5	18
	Lentil Salad with Sherry Vinegar and Mirepoix (NO TURKEY) (p. 192)	89.25	0.5	16.8
	Ice Cream Sandwich (p. 228)	95	5.25	13.4
	Water	0	0	0
TOTALS		1265.75	32.05	150.20

DAY 8

		Cals	Fat G.	Carbs G.
BREAKFAST	Banana Super Yogurt (p. 114)	70	1.6	21
	Granola (p. 116)	56.7	0.2	13.5
	Grapefruit, ½ large	27	0	6.7
	Coffee or green tea	0	0	0
SNACK ONE	Living in Green Smoothie (p. 88)	109.25	0.3	21.25
	Hard-boiled egg, large	78	5.3	0.6
LUNCH	Chopped Salad with Shrimp (p. 182)	98	1.5	10.5
	Avocado	114	10.5	5.9
	Fruit Punch (p. 84)	7	0	2
SNACK TWO	Autumn Snack Clusters (p. 206)	114	0.5	24.8
	Pear, 1 small (5.8 ounces purchase weight)	86	0.2	22.9
	Water	0	0	0
DINNER	Chicken Teriyaki (p. 146)	199	2	17.25
	Vegetable Fried "Rice" (p. 176)	105	0	23
	Chocolate Mint Thins (p. 222)	55	4	8.5
	Water	0	0	0
TOTALS		1118.95	26.1	177.9

DAY 9

BREAKFAST		Cals	Fat G.	Carbs G.
BREAKFAST	Strawberry Shortcake Crunch (p. 110)	87.5	1.8	17
	Hard-boiled egg, large	78	5.3	0.6
	Strawberries, fresh, ½ cup halves	24	0.2	5.8
	Coffee or green tea	0	0	0
SNACK ONE	Pumpkin Pie Smoothie (p. 90)	59	1.5	11.7
	Apple, 1 medium (7 ounces purchase weight)	93	0.3	24.7
LUNCH	Chopped Shiitake and Noodle Salad (p. 138)	87	0.7	16
	Turkey breast, skinless, store-roasted, 3 ounces	115	0.6	0
	Fruit Punch (p. 84)	7	0	2
SNACK TWO	Iced Cappuccino (p. 82)	5	0.3	16.25
	Chocolate Cookies (3 pieces) (p. 238)	141	8.5	46
	Water	0	0	0
DINNER	Spinach Dumplings with Marinara (p. 172)	126	4.4	18.65
	Heart of Palm and Escarole Salad (p. 188)	123	6	16.3
	Mint Chocolate Chip Flurry (p. 224)	119	7	15
	Water	0	0	0
TOTALS		**1064.50**	**36.6**	**190**

DAY 10

		Cals	Fat G.	Carbs G.
BREAKFAST	Super Scramble (p. 112)	135	2.4	12.7
	Cinnamon Apple Rice Bran Muffin (p. 102)	65	1.85	11
	Banana, 1 medium	105	0.4	27
	Coffee or green tea	0	0	0
SNACK ONE	Turkey Jerky (p. 214)	45	0	1
	Apple, 1 small (6 ounces purchase weight)	80	0.3	21
LUNCH	Grilled Turkey Cutlet with Pear Salad (p. 196)	252	8	14
	Hard-boiled egg, large	78	5.3	0.6
	Fruit Punch (p. 84)	7	0	2
SNACK TWO	Prickly Pear Chamomile Cooler (p. 78)	15	0	4
	Pop Chips Original, 1 ounce	120	4	18
	Water	0	0	0
DINNER	Pumpkin Risotto with Sage (p. 160)	138.5	2.5	24.6
	Open-faced Mushroom Salad (p. 132)	99.25	2.5	17.6
	Tartar of Exotic Fruits (p. 236)	79	1.7	16.25
	Water	0	0	0
TOTALS		**1218.75**	**28.95**	**169.75**

DAY 11

		Cals	Fat G.	Carbs G.
BREAKFAST	Green Eggs and Ham (p. 118)	103	2.25	5.4
	Grapefruit, ½ large	27	0	6.7
	Coffee or green tea	0	0	0
SNACK ONE	Living in Green Smoothie (p. 88)	109.25	0.25	21.25
	Apple, 1 small (6 ounces purchase weight)	80	0.3	21
LUNCH	Salad with Carrot-Ginger Dressing (p. 186)	55	0.4	23
	Grilled chicken breast, skinless, store-cooked, 4 ounces	184	4	0
	Fruit Punch (p. 84)	7	0	2
SNACK TWO	Grilled Sweet Potatoes (p. 216)	147	4	23
	Pop Chips Original, 1 ounce	120	4	18
	Water	0	0	0
DINNER	Chicken with Marinated Bean Sprouts (p. 150)	150	1.3	14.5
	½ avocado	114	10.5	6
	Chocolate Cookies (3 pieces) (p. 238)	141.5	8.5	46
	Chocolate Milk (p. 80)	40.5	2.3	5.75
	Water	0	0	0
TOTALS		1278.50	37.8	192.6

DAY 12

		Cals	Fat G.	Carbs G.
BREAKFAST	Sausage and Egg Breakfast (p. 104)	121	0.75	6
	Grapefruit, ½ large	27	0	6.7
	Gluten-free roll, buttered (p. 212)	115.5	2.4	4.75
	Coffee or green tea	0	0	0
SNACK ONE	Prickly Pear Chamomile Cooler (p. 78)	15	0	4
	Pop Chips Original, 1 ounce	120	4	18
LUNCH	Fresh Pea Salad with Smoked Salmon and Creamy Horseradish Dressing (p. 194)	117	2.5	11.4
	Apple, 1 medium (7 ounces purchase weight)	93	0.3	24.7
SNACK TWO	Chocolate Mint Thins (p. 222)	55	4	8.5
	Chocolate Milk (p. 80)	40.5	2.3	5.75
	Water	0	0	0
DINNER	Chili-rubbed Chicken with Black Bean Salsa (p. 154)	173	1.6	12.6
	½ avocado	114	10.5	6
	Tartar of Exotic Fruits (p. 236)	79	1.7	16.25
	Water	0	0	0
TOTALS		1070	30.05	124.65

DAY 13

		Cals	Fat G.	Carbs G.
BREAKFAST	Cocoa Crispies (p. 96)	97.5	2.3	19.5
	Banana, medium	105	0.4	27
	Coffee or green tea	0	0	0
SNACK ONE	Living in Green Smoothie (p. 88)	109.25	0.25	21.25
	Pumpkin seeds, dry-roasted, ¼ ounce	37	3.4	1.2
LUNCH	Creamy Asian-Style Slaw with Salmon (p. 184)	198	7.5	9.6
	Gluten-free roll, buttered (p. 212)	115.5	2.4	4.75
	Water	0	0	0
SNACK TWO	Iced Cappuccino (p. 82)	5	0	16.25
	Coconut Clusters (p. 226)	91	5	14
	Water	0	0	0
DINNER	Soy Spaghetti with Shrimp and Hand-chopped Pomodoro Sauce (p. 168)	185	2.3	16.4
	Heart of Palm Salad (p. 188)	123	6	16
	Ice Cream Sandwich (p. 228)	95	5.25	13.4
	New Year's Resolution Sangria (p. 92)	28.5	0	9
TOTALS		1189.75	34.8	168.35

DAY 14

		Cals	Fat G.	Carbs G.
BREAKFAST	Pancakes with Coconut Nectar (p. 108)	89	0.3	18
	Banana, medium	105	0.4	27
	Hard-boiled egg, large	78	5.3	0.5
	Coffee or green tea	0	0	0
SNACK ONE	Banana Super Yogurt (p. 114)	70	1.5	21
	Granola (p. 116)	56.5	0	13.5
LUNCH	Cream of Mushroom Soup (p. 200)	135	1	31.75
	Gluten-free roll, buttered (p. 212)	115.5	2.4	4.75
	Walnuts, 1 ounce shelled	175	16.7	2.8
	Fruit Punch (p. 84)	7	0	2
SNACK TWO	Pink Lemonade (p. 86)	13	0	4
	Crispy Brown Rice and Wasabi Snack (p. 208)	95	0	22.75
DINNER	Chicken with Parsley, Peppers, and Lemon (p. 152)	194	2	6
	Cauliflower and Kale Salad (p. 190)	43	0.3	9
	Chocolate Mousse (p. 220)	121	7	15.25
	Water	0	0	0
TOTALS		1297	36.9	178.30

Tips:

1. *Look for lettuces, some vegetables, olives, capers, pickled peppers, sprouts, and fresh fruit salad in the supermarket's salad bar and deli departments to help you buy no more than actually necessary and save on pantry space. Be sure to ask if there has been any sugar added to cut fruits, though—that would be a deal breaker.*

2. *Look for nuts, seeds, and coconut products in the bulk-food containers to help you buy no more than you need and save on pantry space.*

3. *You may even be able to find vinegars there as well! Just don't mistake a dressing or vinaigrette for plain balsamic vinegar or red wine vinegar.*

PRODUCE

Vegetables

- ❒ 3 large beets
- ❒ 1 large celery root
- ❒ 3 large parsnips
- ❒ 12 ounces asparagus
- ❒ 2 medium zucchini
- ❒ 2 heaping cups cleaned fresh sugar snap peas
- ❒ 1 small bunch scallions
- ❒ 2 avocados
- ❒ 1 cucumber
- ❒ 5 medium tomatoes
- ❒ 1 (6-inch) firm aloe leaf
- ❒ 1 red jalapeño (green if none available)
- ❒ 6 small sweet potatoes (not yams! White sweet potatoes are acceptable.)

- ❒ ½ head cauliflower, or 1 small head
- ❒ 6 large carrots
- ❒ 6 ounces baby bella (or cremini) mushrooms
- ❒ 5 ounces portabello mushroom (3 ounces after gills are removed)
- ❒ 2 medium onions
- ❒ 2 cups cherry tomatoes
- ❒ 1 head garlic

Lettuces and Herbs

- ❒ 4 bunches fresh basil
- ❒ 1 large bunch fresh cilantro
- ❒ 1 small bunch fresh mint
- ❒ 1 small bunch fresh sage
- ❒ 1 small bunch fresh rosemary
- ❒ 12 ounces spinach (such as Dole), washed
- ❒ ¼ head green cabbage, or 1 very small head, shredded

- [ ] 1 very small bunch Tuscan kale, or 1 pint from salad bar
- [ ] 1 small head escarole, or 4 cups from salad bar
- [ ] 1 romaine heart
- [ ] 1 small head iceberg lettuce, or 4 cups from salad bar
- [ ] 1 large head butter lettuce
- [ ] 1 pint radish sprouts

Fruits and Berries
- [ ] 4 small Pink Lady apples (6 ounces purchase weight)
- [ ] 3 medium Pink Lady apples (7 ounces purchase weight)
- [ ] 2 medium Granny Smith apples (7 ounces purchase weight)
- [ ] 4 medium bananas
- [ ] 1 pint fresh strawberries
- [ ] 3 limes
- [ ] 5 lemons
- [ ] 1 pint fresh pineapple, or ½ cup fresh diced pineapple from salad bar
- [ ] 1 orange in sections
- [ ] 2 large ruby red grapefruits
- [ ] 1 pint fresh fruit salad (citrus, grapes, apples, berries, melon, etc.—check the produce section or salad bar)

Vegetable Blends and Fruit Blends
- [ ] 1 pint pico de gallo (such as Ready Pac)

- [ ] 1 small bottle or bag raw or "live" kimchi (such as Rejuvenate)
- [ ] 1 small bottle or bag "live" sauerkraut (such as Rejuvenate)
- [ ] 1 small container hummus (such as Athenos Original), or ¼ cup from salad bar

FREEZER
- [ ] 1 (10-ounce) box frozen cut corn kernels

DAIRY, DAIRY ALTERNATIVES, AND EGGS
- [ ] 1 pint egg whites (such as Egg Beaters 100% Egg Whites)
- [ ] 6 large eggs
- [ ] 1 small block firm tofu
- [ ] 1 (6-ounce) container plain fat-free Greek yogurt (such as Fage 0%)
- [ ] 1 container 99% plain lactose-free, fat-free kefir (such as Lifeway)
- [ ] 1 ounce Pecorino Romano
- [ ] 1 small container coconut spread (such as Olivio)
- [ ] 1 small bottle virgin coconut oil

BREAD, CRACKERS, AND BAKED GOODS
- [ ] 1 sleeve unsalted brown rice cakes (such as Lundberg)
- [ ] 1 package frozen gluten-free pizza dough (such as Gillian's)
- [ ] 1 package unsalted, gluten-free brown rice thin cakes (such as Suzie's)

PROTEIN

Meat

- ❑ 8 ounces lean ground turkey breast

- ❑ 1 package all-natural, no-nitrate turkey bacon (such as Applegate Farms)

- ❑ 4 ounces boneless skinless chicken thighs, trimmed of all visible fat (3 ounces after trimming)

- ❑ 4 ounces 96% lean ground beef (such as Laura's Lean)

- ❑ 5 ounces pork tenderloin, trimmed of all visible fat (4 ounces after trimming)

Fish

- ❑ 1 (4-ounce) portion cod, haddock, scrod, or hake

- ❑ 6 ounces cooked, peeled, and deveined shrimp

- ❑ 1½ ounces reduced-sodium smoked salmon (such as Trident)

Deli

- ❑ 3 ounces store-roasted pork loin, trimmed of all visible fat, thinly sliced

- ❑ 2 ounces uncured smoked ham (such as Applegate Farms)

- ❑ 2 ounces all natural no-sugar-added smoked turkey breast (such as Applegate Farms)

- ❑ 9 ounces store-roasted skinless turkey breast, thinly sliced

- ❑ 2 slices Canadian bacon (about 1.6 ounces)

DRY GOODS

Legumes

- ❑ 1 bag steamed lentils (such as Melissa's, might be near produce), or 1 can no-salt-added lentils (such as Eden or Bush's)

- ❑ 1 small can no-sugar-added wasabi powder (such as Eden)

- ❑ 1 can reduced-sodium bean chili (such as Amy's)

- ❑ 1 can no-salt-added black beans (such as Eden)

Dried Fruit, Nuts, Seeds

- ❑ 1 (1 ½ -ounce) bag freeze-dried cinnamon-apple crisps (such as Crunchies)

- ❑ 1 (1-ounce) bag Granny Smith apple chips (such as Bare Fruit)

- ❑ 1½ ounces shelled walnuts

- ❑ 6 tablespoons dry-roasted pumpkin seeds (about 2 ounces)

Oil, Vinegar, and Sauces

- ❑ 1 very small bottle balsamic vinegar, or 2 tablespoons from salad bar

- ❑ 1 small bottle Thai-style fish sauce

Coffee and Tea

- ❑ Coffee or green tea (your preference for morning beverage)

- ❑ 1 small box pomegranate tea (such as Yogi)

- ❑ 1 small can unsweetened reduced-fat shredded coconut (such as Let's Do Organic)

- ❑ 1 small box hibiscus tea (such as Teekanne)

- [ ] 1 small box no-sugar-added mixed berry tea (such as Celestial Seasonings Wild Berry Zinger)

OTHER

- [ ] 1 bottle everything bagel spice (such as King Arthur or from a local bagel shop)
- [ ] 1 jar all-natural prune baby food (such as Gerber 1st Foods All Natural)
- [ ] 1 small jar light canola oil mayo (such as Spectrum)
- [ ] 1 hot cherry bomb pepper (such as B&G or check the salad bar), plus 1 teaspoon of its liquid
- [ ] 2 pitted oil-cured black olives (check the salad bar)
- [ ] 6 ounces unsalted fat-free chicken stock (such as Kitchen Basics)
- [ ] 1 small bottle no-sugar-added stevia-sweetened ketchup (such as AlternaSweets)

- [ ] 1 small bag gluten-free corn flour (such as Bob's Red Mill)
- [ ] 1 small bag gluten-free oat flour (such as Bob's Red Mill)
- [ ] 1 container gluten-free rice bran (such as EnerG)
- [ ] 1 small jar Dijon mustard
- [ ] 1 package nori paper
- [ ] 1 small can no-sugar-added pumpkin puree (such as Libby's)
- [ ] 5 ounces gluten-free corn spaghetti (such as Mrs. Leeper's)
- [ ] 1 small bottle nonalcoholic bitters (such as Angostura)
- [ ] 1 small bottle nonpareil capers
- [ ] 1 jar real bacon bits (such as Hormel)
- [ ] 1 can water-packed heart of palm

SHOPPING LIST

WEEK TWO

PRODUCE

Vegetables

- ❒ 1½ cups spinach leaves, washed
- ❒ 3 avocados
- ❒ 1 large beet
- ❒ 1 large celery root
- ❒ 2 large parsnips
- ❒ 2 small sweet potatoes, not yams
- ❒ 1 large carrot
- ❒ 1 onion
- ❒ ½ small red onion (or check the salad bar for sliced red onion; you will need 2 tablespoons)
- ❒ 1 small bunch scallions
- ❒ 4 heaping cups trimmed fresh sugar snap peas
- ❒ 1 cucumber
- ❒ 8 pieces fresh okra
- ❒ 1 small head cauliflower
- ❒ 1 (3-inch) piece fresh ginger
- ❒ 1 head garlic
- ❒ 3 jalapeños
- ❒ 1 red jalapeño, if available
- ❒ 2 poblanos
- ❒ 1 very large portabello mushroom (4 ounces, once gills and stem are removed)
- ❒ 4 ounces baby bella (or cremini) mushrooms
- ❒ 8 fresh shiitake mushrooms
- ❒ 1¼ cups store-cut mixed wild mushrooms
- ❒ 1 head baby bok choy (at least 1 cup chopped)
- ❒ 2 oranges
- ❒ ½ butternut squash
- ❒ 6 cherry tomatoes
- ❒ 1 ripe medium tomato
- ❒ 1 (12-inch) firm fresh aloe leaf
- ❒ 1 head broccoli

Lettuces and Herbs

- ❒ 4 bunches fresh basil
- ❒ 2 bunches fresh cilantro
- ❒ 1 small bunch fresh mint leaves (at least 20 good large leaves)
- ❒ 1 small bunch fresh sage
- ❒ 1 small bunch fresh chives
- ❒ 1 small bunch fresh parsley
- ❒ 14 ounces spinach, washed
- ❒ ½ head escarole, or 1 small head, chopped (or 4 cups chopped, from salad bar)
- ❒ ¼ head red cabbage (½ heaping cup chopped)

- ❐ 2 cups arugula
- ❐ 1 romaine heart (or 2 cups chopped, from salad bar)
- ❐ 1 head Belgian endive
- ❐ 1 very small bunch Tuscan kale
- ❐ ½ cup broccoli sprouts (or your favorite variety of sprout)
- ❐ 1 cup mung bean sprouts
- ❐ 1 small head iceberg lettuce (or 4 cups chopped, from salad bar)

Fruits and Berries

- ❐ 5 medium bananas
- ❐ 2 small apples (6 ounces purchase weight)
- ❐ 2 medium apples (7 ounces purchase weight)
- ❐ 3 small pears (5.8 ounces purchase weight)
- ❐ 1 small Asian pear (feel free to substitute another pear if Asian variety is not available)
- ❐ ½ cup fresh strawberries
- ❐ 1 ripe mango (3 ounces flesh needed)
- ❐ 1 ripe papaya (3 ounces flesh needed)
- ❐ 1½ large ruby red grapefruit
- ❐ 5 limes
- ❐ 5 lemons

Vegetable Blends and Fruit Blends

- ❐ 1 pint store-prepared fresh vegetable medley (cabbage, broccoli, cauliflower, peppers, etc.)
- ❐ 1 pint fresh stir-fry vegetable medley (a mix with broccoli, peppers, mushrooms, onions, snap peas, bean sprouts, etc.), chopped into small pieces
- ❐ 1 pint fresh pineapple, chopped
- ❐ 1 pint fresh ready-made pico de gallo (such as Ready Pac)
- ❐ 1 cup fresh fruit salad (citrus, grapes, apples, berries, melon, etc.—check the produce section or salad bar)

DAIRY, DAIRY ALTERNATIVES, AND EGGS

- ❐ 2½ cups plain 99% lactose-free fat-free kefir (such as Lifeway)
- ❐ 1 (6-ounce) plain fat-free Greek yogurt (such as Fage 0%)
- ❐ 7 large eggs
- ❐ 1 (170-gram) container unsweetened cultured coconut milk (such as So Delicious)
- ❐ 1 small block lite soft tofu (such as Nasoya)
- ❐ 1 ounce Parmigiano-Reggiano
- ❐ 1 pint egg whites (such as Egg Beaters 100% Egg Whites)
- ❐ 1 small container coconut spread (such as Olivio)

BREAD, CRACKERS, AND BAKED GOODS

- ❐ 1 pack unsalted brown rice snaps (such as Edward and Sons)
- ❐ 2 unsalted brown rice cakes (such as Lundberg)
- ❐ 3 packages unsalted brown rice thin cakes (such as Suzie's)

PROTEIN

Meat

- ❒ 4 (4-ounce) skinless chicken cutlets

- ❒ 4 ounces extra-lean ground turkey (such as Jennie-O)

- ❒ 4 ounces turkey tenders (about 1 large tender)

Fish

- ❒ 2 ounces cooked, peeled, and deveined shrimp

- ❒ 2 ounces raw, peeled, and deveined domestic white shrimp

- ❒ 2 ounces reduced-sodium smoked salmon (such as Trident)

- ❒ 3 ounces fresh skinless salmon filet (wild if possible)

Deli

- ❒ 3 ounces skinless store-roasted turkey breast, thinly sliced

- ❒ 6½ ounces cooked boneless skinless chicken breast

- ❒ 1 slice all-natural Canadian bacon (such as Applegate Farms)

DRY GOODS

Legumes

- ❒ 1 can no-salt-added black beans (such as Eden)

Dried Fruit, Nuts, Seeds, Snacks

- ❒ 1 steamed chestnut

- ❒ 1 ounce shelled walnuts

- ❒ ¼ cup dry-roasted, shelled pumpkin seeds (about 1¼ ounces)

- ❒ 1 bag freeze-dried strawberries (such as Just Strawberries)

- ❒ 1 bag freeze-dried apples (such as Just Apples)

- ❒ 1 bag crumbled freeze-dried cinnamon-apple crisps (such as Crunchies)

- ❒ 1 bag unsweetened freeze-dried strawberries (such as Crunchies)

- ❒ 3 (1-ounce) bags Pop Chips Original

- ❒ 1 small bag freeze-dried pineapple (such as Nature's All)

- ❒ 1 container gluten-free banana puffs (such as Happy Puffs—look near the baby foods)

Oil, Vinegar, and Sauces

- ❒ 1 small bottle jalapeño hot sauce (such as Tabasco)

- ❒ 1 small bottle Thai-style fish sauce

Coffee and Tea

- ❒ Coffee or green tea (based on your morning preference)

- ❒ 2 bags pure chamomile tea

- ❒ 1 small box pomegranate tea (such as Yogi)

- ❒ 1 small can unsweetened reduced-fat shredded coconut (such as Let's Do Organic)

- ❒ 1 small box hibiscus tea (such as Teekanne)

- ❒ 1 small box no-sugar-added mixed berry tea (such as Celestial Seasonings Wild Berry Zinger)

OTHER

- ❑ 1 small bag chia seeds (or 1 ounce from the bulk containers at your health food store)
- ❑ 1 small can no-sugar-added wasabi powder (such as Eden)
- ❑ 1 small package nori sheets
- ❑ 1 small can no-sugar-added pumpkin puree (such as Libby's)
- ❑ 1 dried shiitake mushroom
- ❑ 3 bags shirataki spaghetti (such as Zero Calorie or Miracle Noodles)
- ❑ 1 can no-sugar-added fat-free marinara sauce
- ❑ 2 bottled hot cherry peppers (such as B&G), chopped, plus 3 teaspoons of their liquid
- ❑ 1 small package instant soy milk powder (such as Now Foods)
- ❑ 1 box gluten-free rice bran (such as EnerG)
- ❑ 1 very small bottle whole juniper berries
- ❑ 1 small box unsalted fat-free chicken stock (such as Kitchen Basics)
- ❑ 1 small bottle salt-free poultry spice (such as Frontier)
- ❑ 1 small bottle arrowroot powder
- ❑ 1 small bottle water-packed roasted red pepper
- ❑ 1 small bottle water-packed artichoke hearts
- ❑ ½ ounce pitted ripe black olives (about 3 tablespoons)
- ❑ 1 small can lite coconut milk (such as Thai Kitchen)
- ❑ 1 package gluten-free soy spaghetti (such as Explore Asia)
- ❑ 1 small bottle nonpareil capers
- ❑ 1 small bottle nonalcoholic bitters (such as Angostura)
- ❑ 1 bag gluten-free oat flour (such as Bob's Red Mill)

THE NEW LOOK OF YOUR KITCHEN PANTRY

Your pantry will begin to take on a new look after you start this plan. Here's an idea of what your pantry and fridge should start to look like. It includes gluten-free, lactose-free, and refined sugar–free foods.

SWEET

- ❐ Stevia powder (such as Stevia in the Raw)-*keep* 1 box on hand

- ❐ Monk fruit powder (such as Monk Fruit in the Raw)-*keep* 1½ boxes on hand

- ❐ Monk fruit and erythritol crystals (such as Lakanto Golden Sweetener)-*keep* 1 bag (235g) on hand

- ❐ Erythritol (such as Wholesome Sweeteners)-*keep* ¼ of a 12-ounce bag on hand

- ❐ Coconut nectar (such as Coconut Secret)-*keep* 1 bottle on hand

- ❐ Coconut crystals (such as Coconut Secret) -*keep* ¼ of a can on hand

- ❐ Stevia-sweetened no-sugar-added dark chocolate (such as Lily's or Lakanto)-*keep* 2 (3-ounce) bars on hand

- ❐ Raw agave nectar-*keep* ¼ of a 6-ounce bottle on hand

SPICES AND SHELF-STABLE DAIRY ALTERNATIVE

- ❐ Pure vanilla extract (such as Frontier or Simply Organic) -*keep* 1 (2-ounce) bottle on hand

- ❐ Unsweetened vanilla almond milk (such as Silk or Almond Breeze)-*keep* 1 32-ounce box on hand

- ❐ 1 can smoked paprika -*keep* ¼ can or bottle on hand

- ❐ 1 can blackening spice (such as Phillips) -*keep* ¼ can or bottle on hand

- ❐ 1 small container whole nutmeg-*keep* ¼ can or bottle on hand

- ❐ 1 small bottle pure peppermint essential oil -*keep* ¼ bottle on hand

- ❐ 1 small bottle ground cinnamon-*keep* ¼ can or bottle on hand

- ❐ 1 small bottle poultry spice-*keep* ¼ can or bottle on hand

- ❐ 1 small bottle arrowroot powder-*keep* ¼ can or bottle on hand

OILS, VINEGARS, SAUCES, DRESSINGS

- ❐ Olive oil cooking spray-*keep* 1 can on hand

- ❐ Extra virgin olive oil-*keep* 1 small 8-ounce bottle on hand

- ❐ White wine vinegar—*keep* ½ of an 8-ounce bottle on hand

- ❐ Sherry wine vinegar—*keep* ¼ of an 8-ounce bottle on hand

- ❐ Gluten-free reduced-sodium tamari (such as San-J)-*keep* ½ of a 10-ounce bottle on hand

- ❐ Unrefined coconut oil-*keep* ¼ cup on hand

DRY GOODS

- ❐ Instant espresso powder (such as Medaglia d' Oro)-*keep* 1 2-ounce bottle on hand

- Egg white powder (such as Jay Robb or Deb El Just Whites)-*keep* 1 12-ounce bag or 2 3-ounce cans on hand

- Puffed brown rice (such as Arrowhead Mills)-*keep* ½ of a 6-ounce bag on hand

- Pysllium Husk (such as Yerba)-*keep* ½ of a 12-ounce container on hand

- Dark cocoa powder, unsweetened-*keep* 1 8-ounce container on hand

- Gluten-free all-purpose flour (such as Glutino)-*keep* ½ of a 16-ounce box on hand

- Pectin (such as Pomona)-*keep* 1 packet on hand

- 1 box unflavored powdered gelatin-*keep* 1 envelope on hand

- Gluten-free baking powder -*keep* ½ box on hand

- Textured vegetable protein-*keep* 2 cups on hand

FROZEN

- 1 loaf gluten-free multigrain bread (such as Udi's; keep frozen and pull out one slice at a time)-*keep* 2 slices on hand

- Strawberries, no sugar added-*keep* 1 16-ounce bag on hand

- Peaches, no sugar added -*keep* 1 16-ounce bag on hand

- No-sugar-added vanilla frozen dessert (such as So Delicious Vanilla Bean) -*keep* 1 pint on hand

Important Recommendations

I'd really like you to establish a baseline prior to beginning the 14-Day Plan. Your weight and health will improve rapidly, so it's a good idea to have evidence of these positive changes. You'll find it rewarding and inspiring to track your progress in ways that can be easily measured. I recommend that you:

- *Weigh yourself on "0" day (the day before Day 1). Write your weight down. Weigh yourself again on Day 5, Day 10, and Day 14. If you still have more weight to lose, continue the diet until you reach your goal.*

- *Note your blood pressure. Take a baseline blood pressure reading, either at your doctor's office, or in one of those pharmacy blood pressure measurement stations (my doctor tells me they are very accurate). Note and record changes, before, during, and after twenty-eight days.*

- *Get a lipid profile. Often when people switch to this type of food plan, there are positive changes in glucose, cholesterol, and triglycerides. Consider having blood tests done prior to beginning the program, and afterward. Your doc can arrange for these tests, or you can schedule them yourself at a reputable lab.*

- *Always check with your health-care provider prior to embarking on this diet, to get his or her approval.*

NOW, LET'S COOK YOUR BUTT OFF!

The next section of the book begins the recipes. All the dishes you're about to make are easy to prepare. I give you information on calorie and fat content (and how these recipes compare to their fattening counterparts before I remade them my way), on prep times, the calorie burn of preparing the recipes, tips, and other important nutrient information.

If you see some unusual ingredients in these recipes or items that you've never purchased before, let me assure you that they are not hard to find; most are available in stores, or if not, they can be found online with a simple search. To help you here, I've listed my favorite brands in the recipes.

So if you're ready, let's turn to the recipe section, head to the kitchen, and start cooking!

CHAPTER 5

Day 15 and Beyond

YOU'VE just completed fourteen days of sugar-free, gluten-free, low-lactose eating—and you've shed unwanted pounds quickly by removing the junk that has blocked your way to trim, healthy living.

Now the question is: Where do you go from here?

The answer is easy. Starting on day 15, every day for the next two weeks, choose a breakfast, lunch, dinner, and three snacks from my recipe list, cook your butt off, and continue to watch more weight fall off. In other words, simply mix and match breakfasts, lunches, dinners, and snacks to get all the fat-burning nutrition you need every day. Try to keep your calories around 1,200 a day for the best results. Here's a meal planner to help you make the right choices:

COOK YOUR BUTT OFF! MEAL PLANNER

DAY 15

MEAL	MEAL CHOICES FROM RECIPE LIST	CALORIES
BREAKFAST		
LUNCH		
DINNER		
SNACKS (3)		
TOTAL CALORIES		

DAY 16

MEAL	MEAL CHOICES FROM RECIPE LIST	CALORIES
BREAKFAST		
LUNCH		
DINNER		
SNACKS (3)		
TOTAL CALORIES		

DAY 17

MEAL	MEAL CHOICES FROM RECIPE LIST	CALORIES
BREAKFAST		
LUNCH		
DINNER		
SNACKS (3)		
TOTAL CALORIES		

DAY 18

MEAL	MEAL CHOICES FROM RECIPE LIST	CALORIES
BREAKFAST		
LUNCH		
DINNER		
SNACKS (3)		
TOTAL CALORIES		

DAY 19

MEAL	MEAL CHOICES FROM RECIPE LIST	CALORIES
BREAKFAST		
LUNCH		
DINNER		
SNACKS (3)		
TOTAL CALORIES		

DAY 20

MEAL	MEAL CHOICES FROM RECIPE LIST	CALORIES
BREAKFAST		
LUNCH		
DINNER		
SNACKS (3)		
TOTAL CALORIES		

DAY 21

MEAL	MEAL CHOICES FROM RECIPE LIST	CALORIES
BREAKFAST		
LUNCH		
DINNER		
SNACKS (3)		
TOTAL CALORIES		

DAY 22

MEAL	MEAL CHOICES FROM RECIPE LIST	CALORIES
BREAKFAST		
LUNCH		
DINNER		
SNACKS (3)		
TOTAL CALORIES		

DAY 23

MEAL	MEAL CHOICES FROM RECIPE LIST	CALORIES
BREAKFAST		
LUNCH		
DINNER		
SNACKS (3)		
TOTAL CALORIES		

DAY 24

MEAL	MEAL CHOICES FROM RECIPE LIST	CALORIES
BREAKFAST		
LUNCH		
DINNER		
SNACKS (3)		
TOTAL CALORIES		

DAY 25

MEAL	MEAL CHOICES FROM RECIPE LIST	CALORIES
BREAKFAST		
LUNCH		
DINNER		
SNACKS (3)		
TOTAL CALORIES		

DAY 26

MEAL	MEAL CHOICES FROM RECIPE LIST	CALORIES
BREAKFAST		
LUNCH		
DINNER		
SNACKS (3)		
TOTAL CALORIES		

DAY 27

MEAL	MEAL CHOICES FROM RECIPE LIST	CALORIES
BREAKFAST		
LUNCH		
DINNER		
SNACKS (3)		
TOTAL CALORIES		

DAY 28

MEAL	MEAL CHOICES FROM RECIPE LIST	CALORIES
BREAKFAST		
LUNCH		
DINNER		
SNACKS (3)		
TOTAL CALORIES		

ON YOUR OWN

Because you've gotten used to cooking and eating this way, I now declare you equipped to alter your favorite recipes on your own to suit your tastes. You'll enjoy creating your own no-sugar, gluten-free, low-lactose, and low-fat recipes, and I'm going to give you an easy tutorial to get you started.

Converting a recipe can be tricky, and it's not an exact science. Start with a couple of your favorite recipes, and make changes to them. It may take you several tries to get the recipe the way you like it. I keep a notebook in my kitchen, recording all my trials, errors, and successes. That way, I can remember what worked and what didn't and can replicate the successes next time. Be patient. It's worth the time—and your health—to get recipes right. Grab your apron, and let's get started.

GETTING OFF SUGAR

Cooking without sugar requires some experimentation, since sugar helps to give baked goods their texture and appealing flavor. As with any modifications, you may need to try the recipe several times before you reach your desired outcome. Here are some suggestions:

- *For natural sweetness, try using fruits in cookies, cakes, quick breads, muffins, pancakes, or waffles. Good choices include pureed apples and bananas.*

- *Try natural (no-sugar-added) fruit juice instead of sugar and liquids such as milk. Add ½ teaspoon baking soda per cup of liquid.*

- *Enhance flavor the calorie-free way with spices (cinnamon, allspice, nutmeg, cloves, etc.) and extracts (vanilla, lemon, almond, and chocolate).*

- *To lighten calories, increase nutrition, and/or reduce the glycemic effect, cook and bake with the sugar alternatives listed below.*

Cooking and Baking with Alternative Sweeteners

An easy way to cut back on calories without feeling deprived is to cook or bake with alternative sweeteners.

RAW AGAVE NECTAR

In recipes, use ¼ to ⅓ cup agave for each 1 cup sugar. In baking, reduce the liquid by 2 tablespoons for each ¼ cup agave used.

COCONUT NECTAR

This sweetener can be used as a replacement for the same amount of sugar in recipes.

ERYTHRITOL

This sweetener can be used as a replacement for the same amount of sugar in recipes.

MONK FRUIT

A product such as Monk Fruit in the Raw converts like this:

1 teaspoon sugar = ½ packet

2 teaspoons sugar = 1 packet

1 tablespoon sugar = 1½ packets

¼ cup sugar = 6 packets

For bulk conversions, this sweetener can be used as a replacement for the same amount of sugar in recipes.

PALM SUGAR

This sweetener can be used as a replacement for half the amount of sugar in recipes.

STEVIA

In baking, use 1½ tablespoons powdered (or 1 teaspoon liquid) for 1 cup sugar.

FREEZE DRIED FRUIT (NO SUGAR ADDED)

Use freeze-dried fruit chopped and pushed through a fine mesh sieve in any application that requires sweetening.

GOING GLUTEN-FREE

Most recipes, even your favorites, can be easily made without gluten.

Converting recipes to gluten-free requires several steps, but is relatively easy. Here are some pointers:

- **Use a gluten-free flour mix.** *These products are easy to find in most supermarkets. A popular flour is Bob's Red Mill all-purpose gluten-free flour.*

- **Forget flour altogether.** *Grind raw almonds in your blender to a flour-like consistency. Finely ground almonds create a delicious, high-fiber flour that can replace wheat flour in a recipe at a 1:1 ratio.*

- **Use xanthan gum.** *It helps the cookies or muffins rise as well as stick together and not be crumbly, tough, or rubbery. Add ¼ teaspoon xanthan gum for each 1 cup flour your recipe calls for. Once xanthan gum is added, gently mix it in the batter or dough, using only 5 to 10 strong strokes. Very little stirring is recommended after that.*

- **Consider arrowroot powder.** *If you can't find xanthan gum, use arrowroot powder instead. As a general rule, use ½ teaspoon arrowroot powder for each 1 cup gluten-free flour called for in a recipe.*

- **Double the baking powder.** *This is because gluten-free baked foods don't rise as well as wheat-based recipes. (By the way, baking soda doesn't work well in gluten-free baking.)*

- **Finally, bake your gluten-free recipe** *at the same temperature and about the same amount of time as the original recipe calls for.*

- **Use psyllium husk instead of flour.** *This is nature's scrub brush and has a unique property that provides elasticity similar to products containing gluten. I use psyllium in recipes such as my crispy tacos (page 130) and my gluten-free roll (page 212).*

TAKE IT DAIRY FREE

Modifying recipes to dairy free is a cinch these days with all the new products available. Some suggestions:

- *Use a dairy-free fats or dairy-free shortenings such as coconut manna and avocado in place of butter or dairy-based margarine.*

- *Replace cow's milk with the dairy-free milk of your choice. Almond, soy, coconut, and rice milk all work fine. If a recipe calls for buttermilk, use 1 to 2 teaspoons rice vinegar to sour the milk substitute you choose.*

- *Substitute soy milk or juice for the milk in a pancake recipe.*

- *Replace butter with almond butter.*

- *Substitute soy cheeses for regular cheeses, and some cheeses are natually low in lactose, like Parmigiano-Reggiano*

LOWER THE LACTOSE WITH YOGURT

As I've mentioned, yogurt is low in lactose and therefore easier on your digestive system. And soy yogurt has no lactose. Both make great substitutes for sour cream, whipped topping, and mayonnaise. Greek yogurt also makes a wonderful substitute for sour cream or toppings. I also like to make yogurt cheese, which has 10 calories per tablespoon when made with low-fat yogurt. Here's how I do it:

Line a colander or strainer with a coffee filter. Fill it with yogurt, set it over a saucepot, and cover with plastic wrap. Place this in your fridge overnight. The next morning, you'll have a lovely soft "cheese." Transfer your "cheese" to a separate container and use it as a base for a tasty dip or spread for breads. You can also use it as a substitute for sour cream or whipped cream.

OUT WITH THE FAT

I use very little added fat in my recipes, preferring to rely more on vegetable cooking sprays. There are other ways to oust the fat, too, without taking away from the flavor or consistency of your dish.

When decreasing fat in baked goods, for example, replace some or all of the fat with an equal amount of one of the following items:

- *Sugar-free apple butter*
- *Organic sugar-free baby food (fruit flavored)*
- *Crushed pineapple*
- *Grated carrots, zucchini, or apples*
- *Mashed bananas*
- *Prune puree or prune butter*
- *Mashed or cooked pumpkin, squash, or yams*
- *Nonfat yogurt*

When you decrease or replace some of the fats in the recipe, use a lower oven temperature for baking in order to preserve moisture. After baking and cooling, refrigerate the items to keep them fresh.

CUT THE CALORIES IN YOUR FAVORITE RECIPES

You can cut the calories, as well as the fat and sugar, in recipes by using egg whites, egg white powder, or an egg substitute for the whole egg. In baking, use two egg whites for the first whole egg and one egg white for each additional egg. If you use an egg substitute product, the container will tell you the exact conversion. Using these subs saves you around 50 calories for each egg substituted.

Love chocolate but hate the calories? Per ounce, baking chocolate adds 140 calories and 15 grams of fat. Try replacing this ingredient with 3 tablespoons unsweetened cocoa powder and 2 teaspoons water. This substitution adds only 45 calories and 5 grams of fat, and it's suitable for cakes, brownies, and puddings.

Some other low-calorie "tricks" to consider are substituting Canadian bacon, turkey bacon, turkey ham, or turkey sausage for regular bacon or sausage. Also, use extra-lean or lean ground beef, chicken, or turkey in place of regular ground beef.

Why not ease back on the amount of meat in recipes, too, in order to cut calories and get more nutrition? Use three times as many vegetables as the meat in soups, stews, casseroles, and on pizza. Experiment with converting recipes such as chili with ground beef to chili with beans. Do the same with tacos or sloppy joes. Skip putting meat in soups, stews, and stir-fried dishes. Replace meat with chunks of tofu (soybean curd), tempeh (fermented soybean curd), or more vegetables. Try meatless sandwich spreads, such as hummus or mashed avocados, or sandwiches made with veggies.

Experiment with new foods. By learning to enjoy a variety of grains, legumes, nut and seed butters, fruits, and vegetables, you'll greatly expand your food repertoire—and bolster your health.

A funny thing will happen when friends and family try your scaled-down versions of familiar recipes. They'll often like the new version better. Imagine their surprise after you reveal what's missing from the recipes. You may just get some converts right on the spot!

Changing to this way of eating need not be overwhelming or daunting. You can do it. And remember, it's more a lifestyle change than a diet. It's about making daily decisions that turn into lifelong choices, and it can be a wonderful journey.

PART TWO

THE RECIPES

CHAPTER 6

Beverage Recipes:

Apple, Lime, and Basil Smash

Prickly Pear Chamomile Cooler

Chocolate Milk

Iced Cappuccino

Fruit Punch

Pink Lemonade with Mint

Living in Green Smoothie

Pumpkin Pie Smoothie

New Year's Resolution Sangria

APPLE, LIME, AND BASIL SMASH

LOOKING FOR another cool way to get your apple a day? Look no further than this refreshing blender drink. The lime-basil match may throw you, but both make the apple flavor pop. This beverage makes a great low-calorie snack and a thirst-quenching drink on a hot day.

Yield	Prep time	Processing time	Calorie Burn	Calories	Net-Calories
1 (16-ounce) beverage	approximately 5 minutes	approximately 10 minutes	65	37	-28

Ingredients:

1	cup cold water
1	tablespoon fresh lime juice
1	packet stevia extract (such as Stevia in the Raw)
¼	cup fresh basil, plus 1 sprig to garnish
⅛	teaspoon grated lime zest
1	small Granny Smith apple
1	cup ice cubes
1	lime slice, to garnish

Method:

1. Pour the water, lime juice, and stevia in a bowl, set aside. Place basil and lime zest into a mortar and smash into a fine paste with the pestle, then add the paste to the water mixture.
2. Using a Microplane, grate the apple into a puree over a plate. You'll need ½ cup of grated apple. Add the puree to the water mixture and mix with a spoon.
3. Place the ice into a large clean kitchen towel, and using a meat mallet or cast-iron pan, smash it into little pieces. Spoon the ice evenly into a pint-sized mason jar, add the apple mixture, screw the lid on tightly, and shake for at least 1 minute. Garnish with a lime wedge and basil sprig.

Per serving:

37 calories, 0.1g fat (0g sat), 0mg cholesterol, 1mg sodium, 10.25g carbohydrate, 1.6g fiber, 0.3g protein

Recommended Ready-Made Version:

Stevita Lime Stick Mix
Fat: 0g / Calories: 0 cal

BEFORE

120 | **0**

Calories | Fat

AFTER

37 | **0**

Calories | Fat

fitbit food log SCAN HERE

PRICKLY PEAR CHAMOMILE COOLER

THE HERB CHAMOMILE is loaded with health perks: It calms frayed nerves and helps you sleep; eases an upset tummy, and soothes coughs and colds. Here, I've used it in a beverage that tastes better than any high-sugar fruit tea anywhere. The resulting drink is practically zero calories, thanks to the addition of applesauce and stevia, so enjoy it to your heart's content.

Yield	Prep time	Processing time	Calorie Burn	Calories	Net-Calories
1 (16-ounce) beverage	approximately 5 minutes	approximately 10 minutes	65	15	-50

Ingredients:

1 cup cold water

2 bags organic chamomile tea (such as Stash)

½ juniper berry, smashed

1 cup crushed or small cubes of ice, plus more for serving

1 medium pear, the riper the better

4 packets monk fruit extract (such as Monk Fruit in the Raw)

2 teaspoons erythritol (such as Wholesome Sweeteners)

½ teaspoon fresh lemon juice

1 thin slice jalapeño

Method:

1. Put the water, tea, and juniper berry into a wide saucepan and cover. Bring to a boil over medium-high heat, then reduce the heat to maintain a simmer, about 2 minutes. Gently press the tea bags to extract the flavor but do not break them open.

2. Place the ice in a large bowl and pour the hot tea over the ice. Stir until cooled. Remove the tea bags and juniper and press out any remaining liquid. Grate the pear into a puree with a Microplane onto a plate. You will need ¼ cup of the puree.

3. Place the strained tea, monk fruit, erythritol, lemon juice, jalapeño, and grated pear into a pint-sized mason jar. Place the lid on the jar and shake vigorously until everything is well mixed. Open the jar, add ice to fill to the top, and serve.

Per serving:

15 calories, 0g fat (0g sat), 0mg cholesterol, 5mg sodium, 4.25g carbohydrate, 0.375g fiber, 0.1g protein

Recommended Ready-Made Version:

Lipton Diet Green Tea
Fat: 0g / Calories: 0 cal

BEFORE

200 | 0

Calories | **Fat**

AFTER

15 | 0

Calories | **Fat**

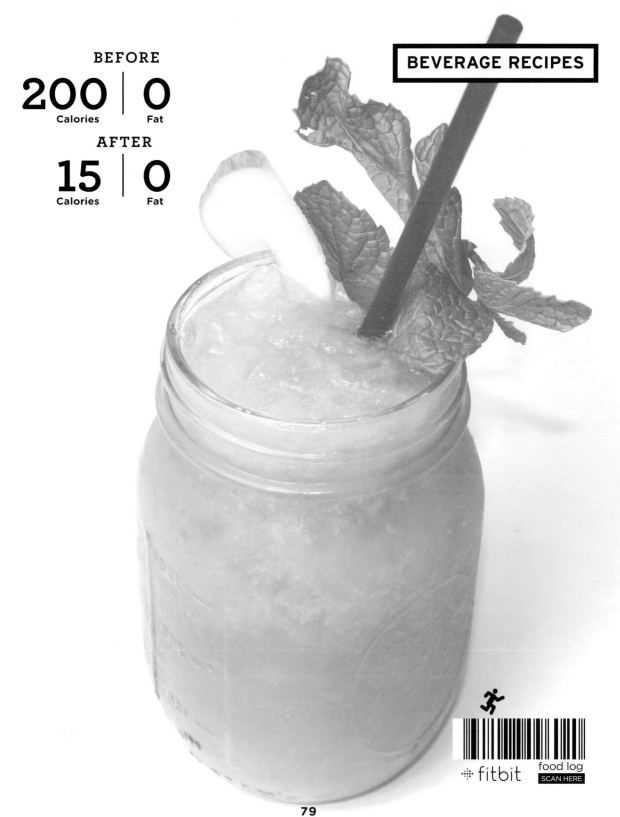

fitbit **food log** SCAN HERE

COOK YOUR BUTT OFF!

CHOCOLATE MILK

HERE'S SOMETHING that brings on flashes of pure childhood goodness: chocolate milk. For this version, I've substituted unsweetened almond milk for cow's milk. It's a great swap, since both beverages have roughly the same amount of protein, 7 to 8 grams. Unsweetened almond milk is much lower in sugar (5 grams) compared to 12 grams in cow's milk. With the addition of dark cocoa and natural sweeteners, they taste similar, too. Note that my version delivers only 10 percent of the calories in the original. There's a secret ingredient here, too: aloe juice, the healing juice of aloe leaves that is so kind to your digestive system. It makes a perfect—and natural—thickener that adds a rich and silky texture to this beverage.

Yield	Prep time	Processing time	Calorie Burn	Calories	Net-Calories
1 (8-ounce) beverage	approximately 8 minutes	approximately 8 minutes	76	40.5	-35

Ingredients:

¾   cup cold unsweetened vanilla almond milk (such as Silk)

¼   cup fresh aloe (fresh aloe is widely available in supermarkets and from florists. Simply look for big healthy green leaves, peel the tough green layer off to reveal the clear usable gel)

3   packets stevia powder (such as Stevia in the Raw)

2   packets monk fruit powder (such as Monk Fruit in the Raw)

⅛   teaspoon kosher salt

1   tablespoon unsweetened cocoa powder

Method:

1. Pour the almond milk into a 16-ounce mason jar and add the aloe gel. Add the stevia, monk fruit, and salt.
2. Working quickly, add the cocoa to the jar and tightly cover the jar. Shake the jar vigorously until everything has dissolved well and there are no visible clumps of cocoa powder.
3. Strain if necessary.

Per serving:

40.5 calories, 2.375g fat (0g sat), 2.25mg cholesterol, 185mg sodium, 5.75g carbohydrate, 2.75g fiber, 1.75g protein

Recommended Ready-Made Version:

So Delicious Chocolate Milk, So Delicious Chocolate Coconut Milk Single
Fat: 5g / Calories: 90 cal

BEFORE

414 | 16.9
Calories | **Fat**

AFTER

40.5 | 2.5
Calories | **Fat**

COOK YOUR BUTT OFF!

ICED CAPPUCCINO

NO BARISTA IN SIGHT? No problem—you can use this foamy almond milk to make some of your favorite coffee bar beverages. This cappuccino will satisfy both your sweet tooth and coffee fix. I am calling for cold water instant espresso powder in this recipe but if you want to use a fresh hot espresso or café Americano then go for it. The foam is stable enough to use for both hot and cold beverages.

Yield	Prep time	Processing time	Calorie Burn	Calories	Net-Calories
1 (10-ounce) beverage	approximately 4 minutes	approximately 10 minutes	89	5	-84

Ingredients:

1	cup plus 2 tablespoons cold water
2½	teaspoons instant espresso powder (such as Medaglia d'Oro)
4	teaspoons monk fruit crystals (such as Lakanto Golden Sweetener)
2	tablespoons unsweetened vanilla almond milk (such as Almond Breeze)
¼	teaspoon egg white powder (such as Deb El Just Whites)
	Cinnamon, for serving

Method:

1. Pour the water into a large bowl with the espresso powder and 3 teaspoons of the monk fruit crystals; stir to dissolve.
2. Place the remaining monk fruit crystals, the almond milk, and the egg white powder in a separate bowl and whisk vigorously until foamy, 1 to 2 minutes.
3. Pour the coffee into a 12-ounce glass filled with ice and spoon the foamed milk evenly on top. Sprinkle with cinnamon and serve.

Tips:

- Add 1 packet of monk fruit extract (such as Monk Fruit in the Raw) to the beginning stage of the milk foam for a sweeter foam and 0 calories, if you have a liking for things a little sweeter.
- For a super-stable milk foam, add a sprinkle (barely $\frac{1}{16}$ teaspoon) gum to the egg white powder when you make the foam.

Per serving:

5 calories, 0.3g fat (0g sat), 0mg cholesterol, 28.75mg sodium, 16.25g carbohydrate, 0.125g fiber, 0.5g protein

Recommended Ready-Made Version:

Starbucks Low Calorie Iced Coffee + Milk
Fat: 0.5g / Calories: 50 cal

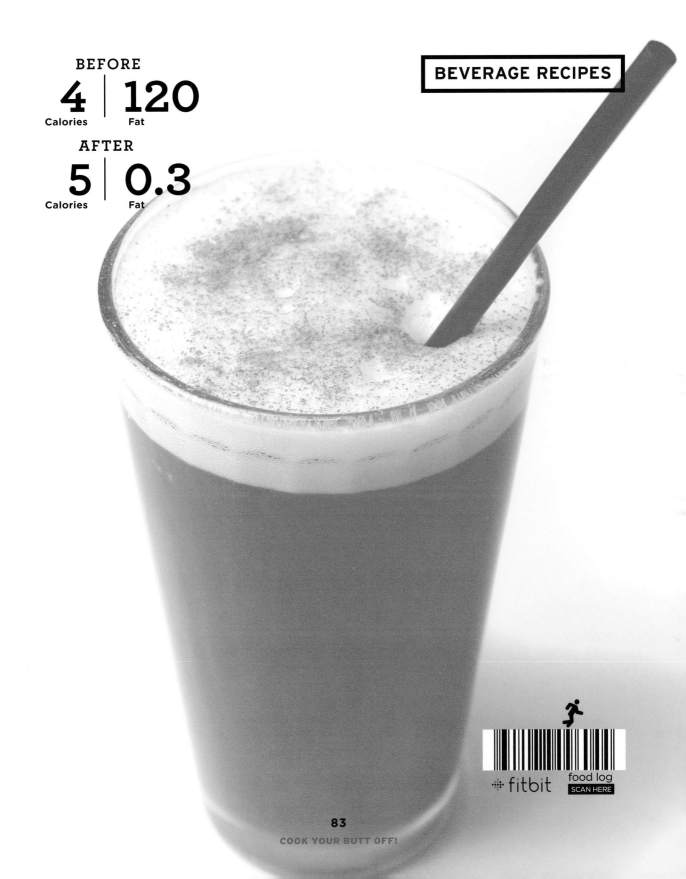

BEFORE

4 | **120**
Calories | Fat

AFTER

5 | **0.3**
Calories | Fat

fitbit food log SCAN HERE

FRUIT PUNCH

KIDS THESE days are drinking too many fruity drinks, which contain far more sugar than fruit, and this habit is probably contributing to the childhood obesity epidemic. I concocted my own version of fruit punch and tested it with the toughest critics I could find: a panel of eight-year-olds. They passed it with flying colors and wanted their cups refilled. So Mom, forget the commercial stuff and serve this instead. Adults will love it, too, since I've removed all those sinful sugary calories but maintained the fruity flavor.

Yield	Prep time	Processing time	Calorie Burn	Calories	Net-Calories
1 beverage	approximately 8 minutes	approximately 10 minutes	52	7	-45

Ingredients:

1	cup water
2	bags wild berry tea (such as Celestial Seasonings Wild Berry Zinger)
1	tablespoon grated pineapple (or crushed pineapple canned in its own juice, drained)
1½	heaping cups ice
1	packet monk fruit extract (such as Monk Fruit in the Raw)
1	packet stevia extract (such as Stevia in the Raw)
½	tablespoon fresh lemon juice

Method:

1. Pour the water into a wide saucepan, add the tea, and place it over high heat. Add the grated pineapple to the pan and bring to a simmer.
2. Place the ice in a large bowl and strain the liquid through a fine-mesh sieve over the ice. Discard the solids in the strainer and stir the liquid until chilled.
3. Stir in the monk fruit, stevia, and lemon juice. Pour evenly into a glass half filled with ice, and serve.

Tip:

Depending on the ripeness of the pineapple, you may need to add more or less sweetener to compensate.

Per serving:

7 calories, 0g fat (0g sat), 0mg cholesterol, 0mg sodium, 2g carbohydrate, .175g fiber, .075g protein

Recommended Ready-Made Version:

Hanson's Natural Fruit Punch Stix
Fat: 0g / Calories: 5 cal

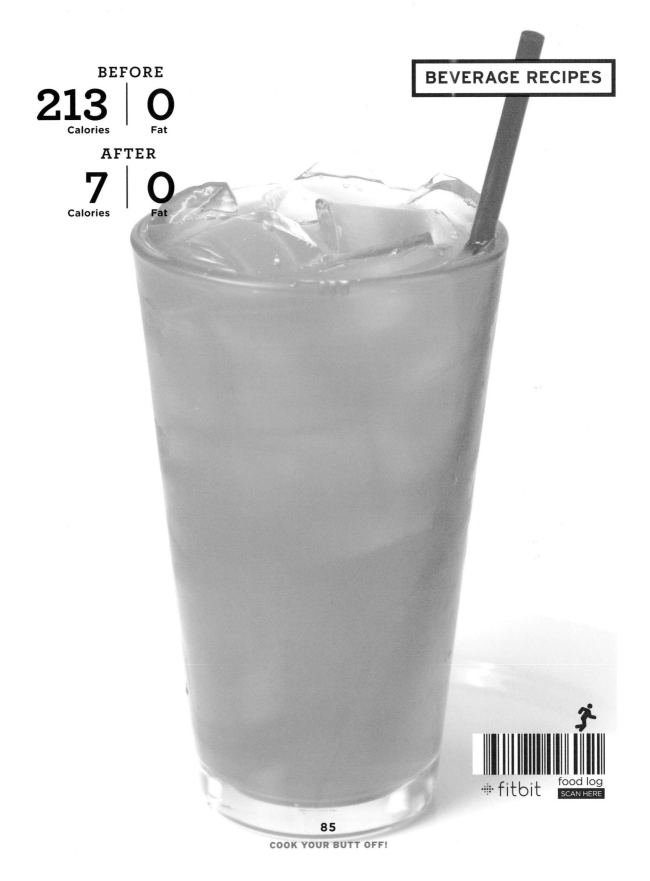

BEFORE

213 | **0**
Calories | Fat

AFTER

7 | **0**
Calories | Fat

fitbit food log SCAN HERE

PINK LEMONADE WITH MINT

ACCORDING TO legend, pink lemonade was created by accident in Texas in 1857. A high-wire circus performer washed her red tights in a vat of lemonade that had been prepared for circus goers. The tights left a red residue that turned the lemonade pink. The circus decided to sell it anyway, promoting it as "pink lemonade." It sold so well that the circus used coloring in subsequent batches and thus created a popular beverage. Unlike that pink lemonade and modern versions, my recipe contains no artificial colorings and is extremely low in calories. Stir up a batch the next time you're thirsty for something sweet and fruity. Although this recipe is for a single serving, I encourage you to make it in large batches. I must mention that this recipe will save you tons of calories if you are accustomed to drinking sugar-sweetened beverages, and it will save your body from aspartame if you are in the habit of drinking diet beverages.

Yield	Prep time	Processing time	Calorie Burn	Calories	Net-Calories
1 (16-ounce) beverage	approximately 10 minutes	approximately 9 minutes	98	13	-85

Ingredients:

1	pint cold water
2	no-sugar-added frozen whole strawberries (such as Dole), grated (1 tablespoon)
⅛	teaspoon grated lemon zest
2	large fresh mint leaves, plus 1 fresh mint sprig for serving
1	tablespoon plus 2 teaspoons strained fresh lemon juice
5	packets monk fruit extract (such as Monk Fruit in the Raw)
	Lemon slice, for garnish

Method:

1. Pour the water into a large bowl. Add the grated strawberries to the water.
2. Place the lemon zest and mint leaves in a mortar and using the pestle, smash into a fine puree. Add the lemon zest mixture to the water along with the lemon juice and monk fruit. Mix well with a whisk to break up all the ingredients.
3. Pour the lemonade into a 20-ounce glass over ice and serve with a mint sprig and a slice of lemon.

Tip:

Simply chop the lemon zest and mint together with a chef's knife if you don't have a mortar and pestle.

Per serving:

13 calories, 0g fat (0g sat), 0mg cholesterol, 0.5mg sodium, 4g carbohydrate, 0.55g fiber, .25g protein

Recommended Ready-Made Version:

NOW Foods Sugar Free Açai Lemonade Slender Sticks
Fat: 0g / Calories: 15 cal

BEFORE

210 | **0**
Calories | Fat

AFTER

13 | **0**
Calories | Fat

fitbit food log
SCAN HERE

COOK YOUR BUTT OFF!

LIVING IN GREEN SMOOTHIE

CREATING A super-green smoothie was a challenge and, I'll admit, a bit daunting. But in the end, I realized that I could have practically a whole day's worth of veggies in one glass. If you have the time, I would recommend quickly wilting half of the spinach in this recipe in a dry pan before using it together with the raw spinach. Both raw and cooked spinach offer different nutrients your body can use. Not a bad deal, right? Besides the green veggie boost, you're getting a microbiotic boost, too, from the kefir. Look for the 99 percent lactose-free varieties to avoid allergic reactions. The addition of basil really smoothes out the other flavors. This makes a very cool and tasty drink.

Yield	Prep time	Processing time	Calorie Burn	Calories	Net-Calories
1 smoothie	approximately 2 minutes	approximately 3 minutes	92	109.25	17

Ingredients:

1½	cups cleaned spinach leaves
½	cup plain 99% lactose-free, fat-free kefir (such as Lifeway)
¾	cup no-added-sugar frozen peaches
5	packets monk fruit extract (such as Monk Fruit in the Raw)
⅛	teaspoon kosher salt
½	heaping cup fresh basil leaves
1	cup ice

Method:

1. Place half the spinach in a large nonstick pan and cook over medium-high heat, stirring, until wilted. Remove from the pan and place on a plate in the freezer to cool.
2. Place the kefir, peaches, remaining raw spinach, monk fruit, and salt in a blender and blend until smooth, about 30 seconds.
3. Remove the cooled wilted spinach from the freezer and add it to the blender. Add the basil leaves and blend until smooth, about 30 seconds. Add the ice and blend until smooth. Pour the smoothie into a glass and serve.

Tip:

Try adding a teaspoon of grated ginger to the recipe for added zing.

Per serving:

109.25 calories, 0.25g fat (0g sat, 0g mono, 0g poly), 2.5mg cholesterol, 96mg sodium, 21.3g carbohydrate, 2g fiber, 7.65g protein

Recommended Ready-Made Version:

Naked Green Machine
Fat: 0g / Calories: 140 cal

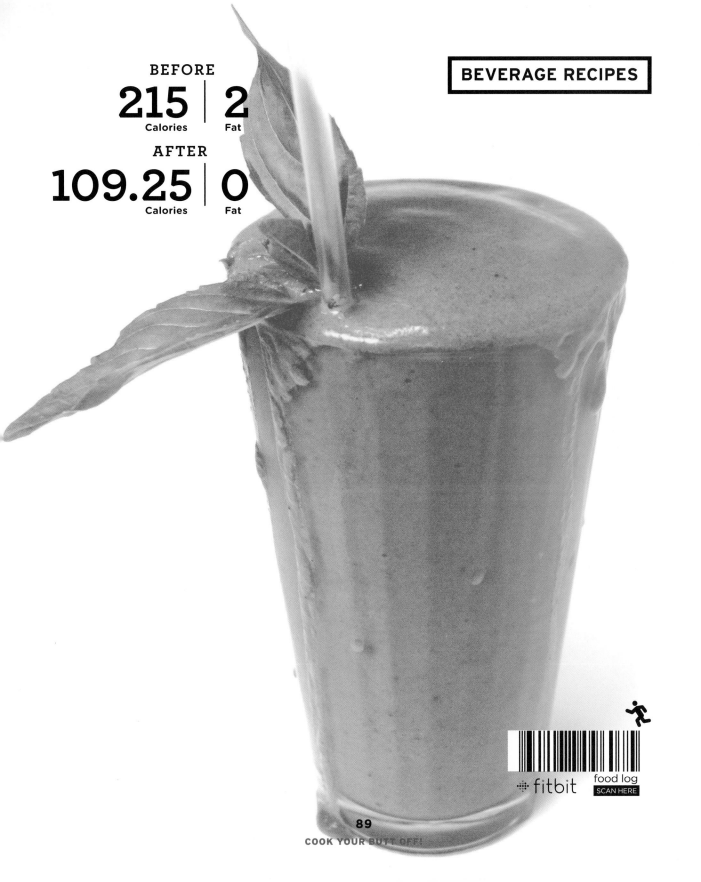

BEFORE
215 | **2**
Calories | Fat

AFTER
109.25 | **0**
Calories | Fat

fitbit food log SCAN HERE

PUMPKIN PIE SMOOTHIE

I'VE BEEN experimenting with lots of dairy-free recipes lately, especially smoothies. This smoothie is one of the results of my experiments. It is easy to make, plus contains vitamin A for healthy skin and eyes, good immune function, and free-radical protection. If you love pumpkin pie, you'll love my pie-in-a-glass version. And no blender necessary!

Yield	Prep time	Processing time	Calorie Burn	Calories	Net-Calories
1 (12-ounce) smoothie	approximately 5 minutes	approximately 10 minutes	67	59	-8

Ingredients:

1	cup cold water
½	cup no-sugar-added pumpkin puree (such as Libby's)
6	packets monk fruit extract (such as Monk Fruit in the Raw)
¼	teaspoon ground cinnamon
½	teaspoon pure vanilla extract
⅛	teaspoon kosher salt
1	tablespoon no-sugar-added vanilla coconut frozen dessert (such as So Delicious)
½	heaping cup ice
1	teaspoon egg white powder

Method:

1. Place the water, pumpkin puree, monk fruit, cinnamon, vanilla extract, salt, and coconut dessert into a cocktail shaker, fasten the lid, and shake vigorously until smooth, about 2 minutes.
2. Place the ice in a clean kitchen towel and smash with a meat mallet until pulverized and powdery but still frozen. Add the crushed ice and egg white powder to the shaker. Shake until smooth and icy, about 1 minute more. Pour into a glass and serve.

Per serving:

59 calories, 1.5g fat (0g sat), 0mg cholesterol, 50mg sodium, 11.7g carbohydrate, 6.55g fiber, 3.6g protein

Recommended Ready-Made Version:

Pure Protein Vanilla Cream Shake
Fat: 0.5g / Calories: 170 cal

BEFORE

790 | **40**

Calories | Fat

AFTER

59 | **1.5**

Calories | Fat

NEW YEAR'S RESOLUTION SANGRIA

IF YOU'RE ready to detox your body from the boozy onslaught of the holidays, try my alcohol-free sangria, based on the popular Spanish fruit and wine punch. The sangria's sweetness and hint of fruity flavors comes from two good-for-you teas. One is pomegranate tea. I've always liked pomegranates, but my love affair with them has been on and off at best. The whole getting-the-seeds-out-before-eating routine makes them tough to enjoy in their raw state. So when all these great pomegranate products came on the market—from juice to tea—I was elated. The tea is rich in health-building antioxidants, and thus very healing. I've also added hibiscus and rose hip tea. Flowering plants are famous for their medicinal properties, and hibiscus is a great example. Medical research indicates that hibiscus tea, in particular, may be helpful in fighting mild to moderately high blood pressure.

Yield	Prep time	Processing time	Calorie Burn	Calories	Net-Calories
1 beverage	approximately 5 minutes	approximately 12 minutes	42	28.5	-13.5

Ingredients:

1	bag pomegranate tea (such as Yogi)
1	bag hibiscus and rose hip tea (such as Teekanne)
¾	cup water
1½	packets monk fruit extract (such as Monk Fruit in the Raw)
6	tablespoons no-sugar-added fresh fruit salad (citrus, grapes, apples, berries, melon, etc.—check the produce section or salad bar at your supermarket), chopped
¼	teaspoon nonalcoholic bitters (such as Angostura)
1	sprig fresh mint, to garnish (optional)

Method:

1. Place the tea bags in a small saucepan and add the water. Cook over medium-high heat until it comes to a simmer, about 2 minutes. Pour the tea through a strainer into a stainless-steel bowl while gently pushing on the tea bags to extract all of the liquid possible.
2. Place the bowl over another bowl filled with ice water and allow the tea to chill, about 3 minutes. Once cool, add the monk fruit, fruit salad, and bitters to the strained tea.
3. Fill a rocks glass one-third of the way with ice, pour the sangria into the glass, and garnish with a sprig of mint partly submerged in the drink.

Tip:

Strain the fruit out of this sangria and place the liquid into a beverage carbonator (I like the Twist'n Sparkle by iSi) for added sparkle, to make the coolest sangria on the block!

Per serving:

28.5 calories, 0g fat (0g sat, 0g mono, 0g poly), 47mg cholesterol, 20.25mg sodium, 9.13g carbohydrate, .6g fiber, 1.9g protein

Recommended Ready-Made Version:

Hanson's Natural Fruit Punch Stix
Fat: 0g / Calories: 5 cal

BEFORE

170 | **0.7**
Calories | Fat

AFTER

28.5 | **0**
Calories | Fat

93
COOK YOUR BUTT OFF!

Cocoa Crispies

Greek Scramble with Tomatoes and Mint

Italian Zucchini Scramble
with Tomatoes and Basil

Cinnamon Apple Rice Bran Muffins

Sausage and Egg Breakfast

Smoked Salmon and Yogurt Breakfast
with Brown Rice Everything Crisps

Pancakes with Coconut Nectar
and Berries

CHAPTER 7

Breakfast Recipes

Strawberry Shortcake Crunch

Super Scramble

Banana Super Yogurt

Fat-free, No-Sugar-Added Gluten-free Granola

Green Eggs and Ham

COCOA CRISPIES

ARE YOUR kiddos clamoring for sugary cereals? How are you responding? I have an idea: Serve my version of those popular cocoa-coated cereals. It's healthy, delicious, and has half the calories of its counterparts. Those commercial cereals are bad for children because they promote bad nutrition and obesity. Both you and your kids will love this recipe, which uses vitamin-rich almond milk. Although growing in popularity, almond milk has been around for centuries. It was developed in the Middle East, where lack of refrigeration made it impossible to keep cow's milk safe for very long.

Yield	Prep time	Processing time	Calorie Burn	Calories	Net-Calories
1 bowl of cereal	approximately 2 minutes	approximately 5 minutes	51	97.5	46.5

Ingredients:
- ¾ cup unsweetened chocolate almond milk (such as Almond Breeze)
- 1 packet stevia powder (such as Stevia in the Raw)
- 2 teaspoons erythritol (such as Wholesome Sweeteners)
- ¾ tablespoon unsweetened cocoa powder (such as Hershey's Special Dark)
- Kosher salt
- ⅓ piece brown rice cake (such as Lundberg; about 7 grams)
- ¾ cup puffed brown rice (such as Arrowhead Mills)

Method:
1. Combine the almond milk, stevia, erythritol, and cocoa with a pinch of salt in a mason jar and shake until all the ingredients are completely dissolved, about 1 minute.
2. Smash the rice cake with a meat mallet until it crumbles into small raisin-sized pieces and mix with the puffed rice. Pour the rice mixture into a bowl, pour the chocolate milk over the top, and serve.

Tip:
You can shake up the milk in a covered container with a tight-fitting lid, make it in batches, and keep it in the refrigerator for easy use during the week.

Per serving:
97.5 calories, 2.3g fat (0g sat, 0g mono, 0g poly), 0mg cholesterol, 138.75mg sodium, 19.5g carbohydrate, 2.625g fiber, 2.75g protein

Recommended Ready-Made Version:
Healthwise Cocoa Protein Cereal
Fats: 3g / Calories: 120 cal

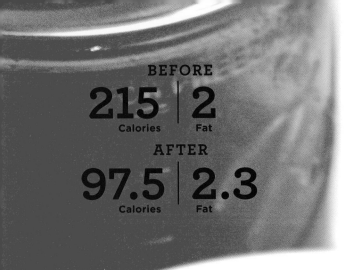

BEFORE

215 | 2
Calories | Fat

AFTER

97.5 | 2.3
Calories | Fat

fitbit food log
SCAN HERE

GREEK SCRAMBLE WITH TOMATOES AND MINT

I LIKE tofu because it absorbs the flavor of anything it's cooked with, from sweet to savory. So I never hesitate to add cubes of tofu to salads, pastas, stir-fry, or creamy desserts. That way, I can create a plant-based dish with through-the-roof flavor. Here, it adds delicious bulk to a delectable egg dish with Grecian flair.

Yield	Prep time	Processing time	Calorie Burn	Calories	Net-Calories
1 breakfast meal	approximately 9 minutes	approximately 10 minutes	49	78.3	29

Ingredients:

6	tablespoons chopped fresh tomatoes
1	tablespoon lightly chopped fresh mint leaves
	Kosher salt and freshly ground black pepper
2	tablespoons firm tofu, drained and crumbled into ¼-inch pieces
1	teaspoon fresh lemon juice
	Olive oil cooking spray
2	ounces washed fresh spinach (such as Dole)
¼	cup egg whites (such as Egg Beaters 100% Egg Whites)

Method:

1. Combine the tomatoes and mint in a small bowl, season with salt and pepper, and set aside. Toss the tofu in a small bowl with a pinch of salt and the lemon juice and set aside.

2. Spray a large nonstick skillet with cooking spray and place it over medium-high heat. Once hot, add the spinach and cook until it is wilted. Press out the water with a spatula and discard the water. Transfer the spinach to a cutting board, chop it into small pieces, and return it to the pan.

3. Vigorously whisk the egg whites until foamy and add them to the pan. Season with salt and pepper, stir to combine with the spinach, and cook until the egg whites are cooked through, about 2 minutes. Transfer the eggs to a plate, top evenly with the tomato mixture and tofu, and serve.

Per serving:

78.3 calories, 1.5g fat (0.325g sat), 2.5mg cholesterol, 161.25mg sodium, 5g carbohydrate, 2.1g fiber, 11g protein

Recommended Ready-Made Version:

Cedarlane Spinach and Mushroom Egg White Omelette
Fat: 12g / Calories: 270 cal

BEFORE

307 | 22.5

Calories | Fat

AFTER

78.3 | 1.5

Calories | Fat

fitbit food log
SCAN HERE

COOK YOUR BUTT OFF!

ITALIAN ZUCCHINI SCRAMBLE WITH TOMATOES AND BASIL

STUDIES SHOW that breakfast is the most skipped meal of the day, with as many as 30 percent of all Americans choosing not to eat it. For someone who loves food as much as I do, intentionally skipping one meal a day—seven a week, fifty-two weeks a year, thousands in an average person's lifetime!—is unfathomable. Come breakfast time, this guy eats. Here's my favorite breakfast in the world, based on what my grandmother used to make for me nearly every Sunday morning when I was a kid. It's loaded with traditional Italian veggies that are high in fat-burning fiber and rich in phytonutrients.

Yield	Prep time	Processing time	Calorie Burn	Calories	Net-Calories
1 breakfast meal	approximately 10 minutes	approximately 5 minutes	52	66	14

Ingredients:

6	tablespoons chopped fresh tomatoes
¼	cup plus 2 tablespoons lightly chopped fresh basil leaves
	Kosher salt and red pepper flakes
	Olive oil cooking spray
½	teaspoon minced garlic
1	cup grated zucchini (grated on the large side of box grater)
¼	cup fresh egg whites, or egg replacement (such as Egg Beaters 100% Egg Whites)

Method:

1. Combine the tomatoes and ¼ cup of the basil in a small bowl, season with salt and red pepper flakes, and set aside.

2. Spray a large nonstick skillet with cooking spray and place it over medium-high heat. Add the garlic and cook, stirring with a wooden spoon, until deep golden brown. Add a pinch of red pepper flakes and remaining 2 tablespoons basil to the pan and cook until the basil has wilted, about 20 seconds. Add the zucchini and cook until it has softened slightly, about 1 minute.

3. Add the egg whites to the pan, season with salt, and cook until the eggs are cooked through, about 2 minutes. Transfer the eggs to a plate, top evenly with the tomato mixture, and serve.

Per serving:

66 calories, 0.525g fat (0.125g sat), 0mg cholesterol, 128mg sodium, 8.5g carbohydrate, 2.3g fiber, 8.3g protein

Recommended Ready-Made Version:

Cedarlane Spinach and Mushroom Egg White Omelette
Fat: 12g / Calories: 270 cal

BEFORE

199 | 10
Calories | Fat

AFTER

66 | 0.5
Calories | Fat

BREAKFAST RECIPES

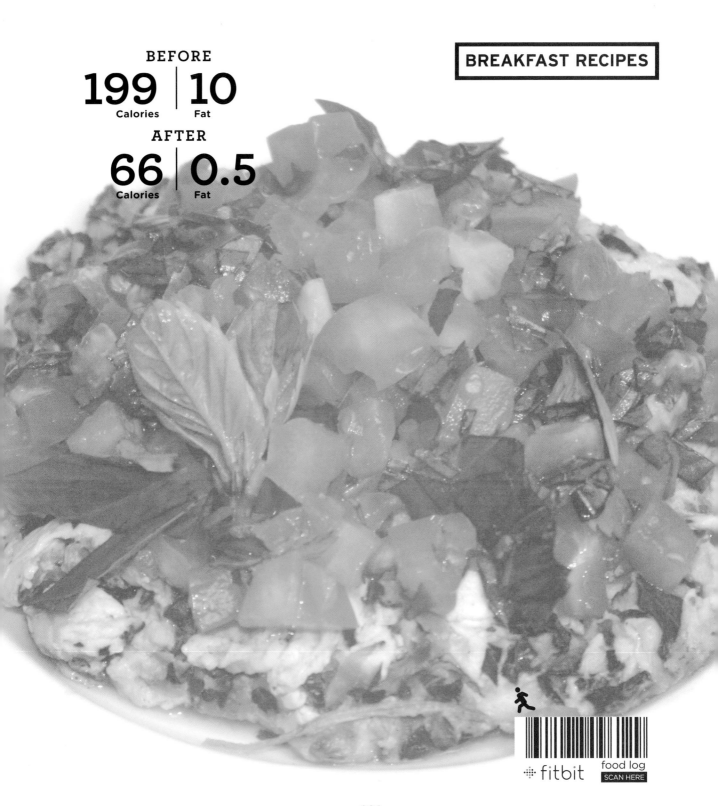

fitbit food log
SCAN HERE

COOK YOUR BUTT OFF!

CINNAMON APPLE RICE BRAN MUFFINS

ALTHOUGH THEY'RE touted as a healthier option than, say, glazed doughnuts, most bran muffins are fattening as hell, loaded with sugar and fat and very little bran. At last I've come up with a recipe that is both good tasting and good for you. Not only is it low in sugar and fat, it is flourless—perfect for those on gluten-free diets. Here it is—enjoy!

Yield	Prep time	Processing time	Calorie Burn	Calories	Net-Calories
1 muffin	approximately 10 minutes	approximately 17 minutes	81	65	-16

Ingredients:

Olive oil cooking spray

2 tablespoons plus 2 teaspoons grated apple (grated on the small holes of box grater, not a zester)

1 teaspoon psyllium husk powder

1⅓ packets monk fruit powder (such as Monk Fruit in the Raw)

⅛ teaspoon kosher salt

⅛ teaspoon ground cinnamon

1 tablespoon rice bran (such as EnerG)

1 tablespoon plus 1 teaspoon egg whites, whipped to soft peaks

Method:

1. Spray an uncoated disposable 12-ounce paper cup with cooking spray, then using a cooking fork or small skewer, poke about 10 holes from the inside out through the bottom of the cup to create vent holes.

2. In a small bowl, whisk together the grated apple and the psyllium with a small whisk until thickened, about 30 seconds. Add the monk fruit, salt, cinnamon, and bran and mix well with a small whisk until smooth. Gently fold the egg whites into the mixture in three additions to keep them fluffy.

3. Spoon the mixture into the prepared cup and microwave on high until set, about 45 seconds. Place the cup on its side and cook for 15 seconds more. Flip the cup to its other side and cook for 15 seconds more. Invert the cup and let the muffin fall out onto a microwave-safe plate and cook for 30 seconds more. Remove and let cool.

Tips:

- You can make these in batches and keep for later.
- Serve with one tablespoon unsweetened Apple Butter for an additional 30 calories.

Per serving:

65 calories, 2g fat (0.3g sat), 70mg cholesterol, 83mg sodium, 11g carbohydrate, 4.65g fiber, 3.75g protein

Recommended Ready-Made Version:

Vitalicious Apple Crumb VitaTops
Fat: 1g / Calories: 100 cal

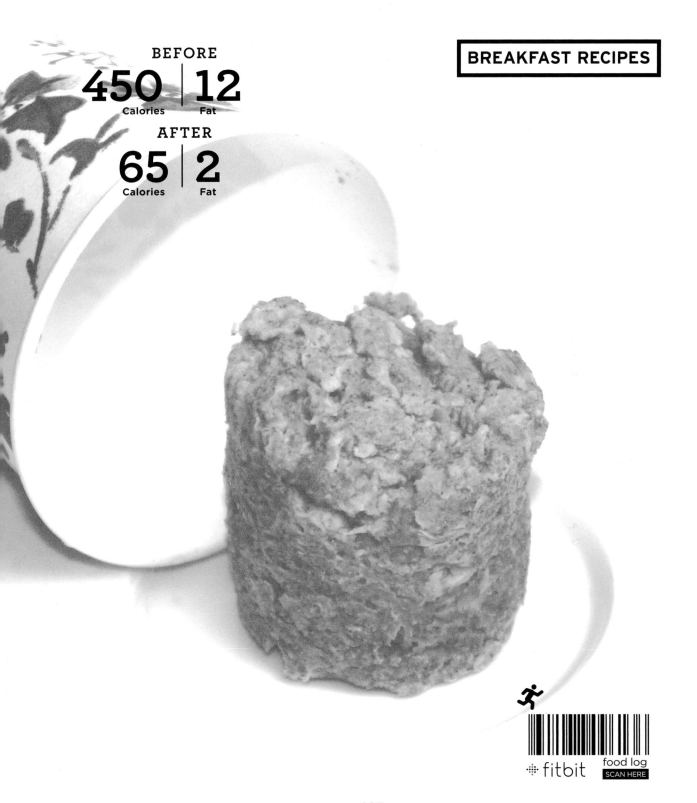

BEFORE

450 | **12**
Calories | Fat

AFTER

65 | **2**
Calories | Fat

fitbit

food log
SCAN HERE

COOK YOUR BUTT OFF!

SAUSAGE AND EGG BREAKFAST

HERE'S A HEARTY dish you'll love. The original tends to be high in fat, however, so I was determined to change it. Plus, all the low-calorie breakfast patties on the shelves are tiny, not very good, and laced with preservatives. Here, I have not only made the patties large and packed with protein, I also hold them together with the added fiber of psyllium husk powder. These patties are super filling and tasty. When served with some scrambled Egg Beaters, you'll be super-fueled for your busy mornings.

Yield	Prep time	Processing time	Calorie Burn	Calories	Net-Calories
1 breakfast meal	approximately 12 minutes	approximately 10 minutes	66	121	55

Ingredients:

Kosher salt and freshly ground black pepper

2 **slices of tomato**

2 **tablespoons cold water**

½ **tablespoon psyllium husk powder**

1 **tablespoon puffed brown rice, chopped**

½ **tablespoon egg white powder**

¼ **teaspoon salt-free poultry spice (such as Frontier)**

2 **ounces extra-lean ground turkey**

Olive oil cooking spray

¼ **cup egg whites (such as Egg Beaters 100% Egg Whites)**

Method:

1. Preheat the oven broiler. Make sure one rack is on the top and one rack is in the middle of the oven. Season the tomato slices with salt and pepper and broil on the top shelf of the broiler until warmed, about 30 seconds. Remove and set aside.

2. Whisk the water and psyllium husk powder in a large bowl until the psyllium has dissolved and the water is thickened, about 1 minute. Add the rice, egg white powder, and poultry spice and mix until dissolved, about 1 minute. Add the turkey and mix until a paste is formed. Season and form into 2 loose mounds.

3. Spray a large nonstick ovenproof skillet with cooking spray and place it over medium-high heat. Add the mounds of turkey and spread them into patties. Cook until starting to brown, about 30 seconds, and then transfer to the oven and cook until patties have cooked through, about 3 to 5 minutes. Remove the pan from the oven, flip the patties, and brown the other side, about 30 seconds. Transfer the patties to a plate.

4. Add the egg whites to the pan, season with salt and pepper, and cook until set, about 2 minutes. Evenly spoon the eggs next to the patties on the plate.

Tips:

This sausage recipe serves well as a blank canvas; try adding crushed fennel seeds or chopped fresh sage for a fresh twist!

Per serving:
121 calories, 0.75g fat (0.25g sat), 27.5mg cholesterol, 193.25mg sodium, 6g carbohydrate, 3g fiber, 21.75g protein

Recommended Ready-Made Version:
Cedarlane Spinach and Mushroom Egg White Omelette
Fat: 12g / Calories: 270 cal

BEFORE
307 | 22.5
Calories | Fat

AFTER
121 | 0.75
Calories | Fat

fitbit food log SCAN HERE

SMOKED SALMON AND YOGURT BREAKFAST WITH BROWN RICE EVERYTHING CRISPS

HERE, I'VE matched microbiota-rich fat-free Greek yogurt with smoked salmon for a delicious low-calorie breakfast that will make your often-tortured bathroom scale send you thank-you notes. Of course, salmon is good and good for you. It's naturally tender, easy to digest, low in bad fat and cholesterol, and loaded with beneficial nutrients and oils. The salmon here is quick to fix—all you have to do is open a package.

Yield	Prep time	Processing time	Calorie Burn	Calories	Net-Calories
1 breakfast meal	approximately 5 minutes	approximately 8 minutes	41	128	77

Ingredients:

Olive oil cooking spray

2 **pieces fat-free, salt-free brown rice crisps (such as Suzie's)**

Kosher salt

½ **teaspoon everything bagel spice (such as King Arthur's)**

1½ **ounces plain fat-free Greek yogurt (such as Fage 0%)**

Cayenne pepper

½ **cup chopped hearts of romaine**

1½ **ounces reduced-sodium smoked salmon (such as Trident), lightly chopped**

Lemon wedge, for serving

Method:

1. Preheat the oven or preheat a toaster oven to 400°F.
2. Place the crisps on a baking sheet and spray with cooking spray. Dust the crisps with salt and everything bagel spice and place in the oven until aromatic and lightly toasted, about 1 minute.
3. Place the yogurt in a bowl and season with salt and a little cayenne. Spoon the yogurt onto a plate and spread it out to cover the bottom of the plate. Evenly distribute the romaine and salmon over the top.
4. Break the crisps into large pieces over the romaine and salmon, letting all the spice and crumbs fall onto the dish, and serve with a wedge of lemon.

Tip:

Try adding a little fresh dill to this recipe or some jalapeño hot sauce for adding zing and less than a calorie.

Per serving:

128 calories, 2.5g fat (0.75g sat), 7.5mg cholesterol, 317mg sodium, 12g carbohydrate, 1.1g fiber, 8.7g protein

BEFORE
800 | **39**
Calories | Fat

AFTER
128 | **2.5**
Calories | Fat

fitbit food log
SCAN HERE

PANCAKES WITH COCONUT NECTAR AND BERRIES

PANCAKES ARE conventionally made with white flour, milk or buttermilk, and vegetable oil. But not these! Mine are gluten-free and dairy free, thanks to the blend of water, egg white powder, psyllium husks, and gluten-free oat flour. For sweetening power, I used cinnamon and low-glycemic coconut nectar. These pancakes are morning comfort food at its best.

Yield	Prep time	Processing time	Calorie Burn	Calories	Net-Calories
1 large pancake or 2 silver-dollar pancakes	approximately 10 minutes	approximately 10 minutes	59	89	29

Ingredients:

- ½ tablespoon coconut nectar
- 4 unsweetened frozen strawberries, thawed
- 3 tablespoons water
- 1 tablespoon egg white powder (such as Deb El Just Whites)
- ½ tablespoon plus ½ teaspoon psyllium husk powder
- ½ tablespoon gluten-free oat flour (such as Bob's Red Mill)
- Kosher salt and ground cinnamon
- Olive oil cooking spray

Method:

1. Combine the coconut nectar and strawberries in a microwave-safe dish, cover with parchment paper, and microwave on high until the berries are warmed through, about 30 seconds. Set aside.
2. Combine the water and egg white powder in large bowl and whisk until fluffy. Add the psyllium, oat flour, and salt and cinnamon to taste and whisk to combine.
3. Spray a large nonstick skillet with cooking spray and place over medium heat. Once the pan is hot add the pancake mix to the pan to make one large or two silver-dollar pancakes. Cook on one side until lightly browned, flip, and continue to cook until browned on the other side and cooked through, about 2 minutes.
4. Place the pancake on a plate and drizzle evenly with the coconut nectar–strawberry mixture.

Tips:

- Add ¼ cup diced, slow-carb green underripe bananas before you flip the pancakes for an additional 18 calories per person with zero added fat!
- Make these pancakes in larger batches, freeze them, and reheat right in your toaster.

Per serving:

89 calories, 0.5g fat (.05g sat), 0mg cholesterol, 90.75mg sodium, 18.14g carbohydrate, 4.6g fiber, 5.33g protein

Recommended Ready-Made Version:

Van's Gluten-free pancakes
Fat: 3g / Calories: 190 cal

BEFORE

230 | **8**

Calories | Fat

AFTER

89 | **0.5**

Calories | Fat

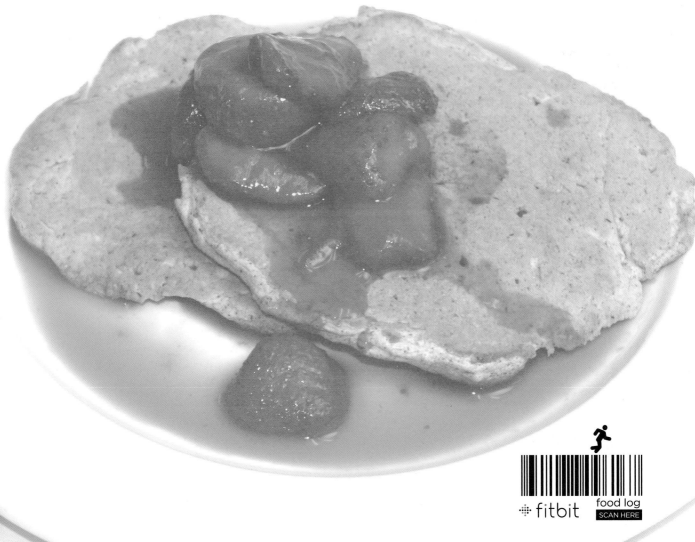

fitbit food log SCAN HERE

STRAWBERRY SHORTCAKE CRUNCH

CAN'T QUITE ditch those sweet cereals? Well, here's a sweet substitute you'll love. It's also gluten free and dairy free—but never free from flavor. Freeze-dried strawberries are my new favorite go-to fruit for zingy taste. And puffed brown rice? Their air virtually puffs out the calories!

Yield	Prep time	Processing time	Calorie Burn	Calories	Net-Calories
1 bowl of cereal	approximately 5 minutes	approximately 5 minutes	56	87.5	31.5

Ingredients:

¾   **cup unsweetened vanilla almond milk (such as Almond Breeze)**
¼   **teaspoon pure natural vanilla extract**
1   **packet monk fruit powder (such as Monk Fruit in the Raw)**
2   **teaspoons erythritol (such as Wholesome Sweeteners)**
    Kosher salt
¼   **cup unsweetened freeze-dried strawberries (such as Crunchies)**
¾   **cup puffed brown rice**

Method:

1. Combine the almond milk, vanilla, monk fruit, erythritol, and a pinch of salt in a small bowl and whisk until all the ingredients have completely dissolved, about 30 seconds.
2. Place two-thirds of the strawberries on a cutting board and chop until they are pulverized. Toss the puffed rice, pulverized strawberries, and remaining strawberries in a bowl to combine. Pour the almond milk mixture over the top and serve.

Tips:

- You can mix the strawberries and rice together and keep in a covered container with a tight-fitting lid, make it in batches, and keep in the pantry for easy use during the week.
- Use another type of nondairy milk if almond is an issue.

Per serving:

87.5 calories, 2g fat (0g sat, 0g mono, 0g poly), 0mg cholesterol, 135mg sodium, 17g carbohydrate, 4.1g fiber, 1.5g protein

Recommended Ready-Made Version:

Barbara's Multigrain Puffin Puffs
Fat: 0g / Calories: 130 cal

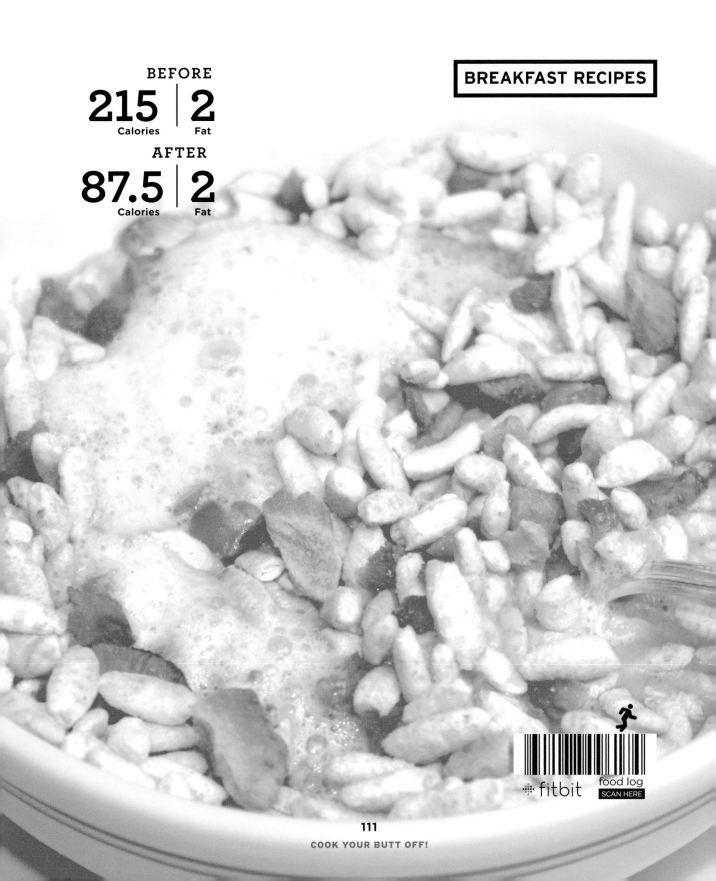

BEFORE
215 | **2**
Calories | Fat

AFTER
87.5 | **2**
Calories | Fat

fitbit food log
SCAN HERE

SUPER SCRAMBLE

I NORMALLY love smoothies for breakfast, but sometimes, they get old. Here's a dish that's just as quick to fix. It's high in protein (over 21 grams in a serving), with less then 3 grams of fat, thanks to the combo of soy milk powder, chicken breasts, and egg whites. Top it with pico de gallo for an extra flavor blast.

Yield	Prep time	Processing time	Calorie Burn	Calories	Net-Calories
1 breakfast meal	approximately 10 minutes	approximately 5 minutes	58	135	77

Ingredients:

2   tablespoons cold water
¼   cup egg whites (such as Egg Beaters 100% Egg Whites)
1   tablespoon soy milk powder (such as NOW Foods)
1   tablespoon egg white powder (such as Deb El Just Whites)
     Kosher salt and freshly ground black pepper
     Olive oil cooking spray
6   tablespoons fresh ready-made pico de gallo (such as Ready Pac)
¼   cup diced cooked boneless skinless chicken breast

Method:

1. Combine the water and egg whites in a small bowl and whisk in the soy milk powder and egg white powder until smooth, about 30 seconds. Season with salt and pepper.
2. Spray a nonstick skillet with cooking spray and place it over medium-high heat. Once the skillet is hot, add the egg mixture and cook, stirring with a rubber spatula, until the egg whites are just about cooked, about 2 minutes. Turn off the heat and let them finish cooking in one even layer, about 1 minute. In a small bowl, mix the pico de gallo with the chicken and season with salt and pepper.
3. Fold the eggs like an omelet on a plate and spoon the chicken and tomato mixture over the top.

Tip:

Serve with a lime wedge, cilantro, and hot sauce for next to no added calories and a real zippy way to greet your day.

Per serving:

135 calories, 2.5g fat (0.5g sat), 2.25mg cholesterol, 333.5mg sodium, 12.7g carbohydrate, 0.5g fiber, 21.85g protein

Recommended Ready-Made Version:

Cedarlane Spinach and Mushroom Egg White Omelette
Fat: 12g / Calories: 270 cal

BEFORE

674 | 51
Calories | Fat

AFTER

135 | 2.5
Calories | Fat

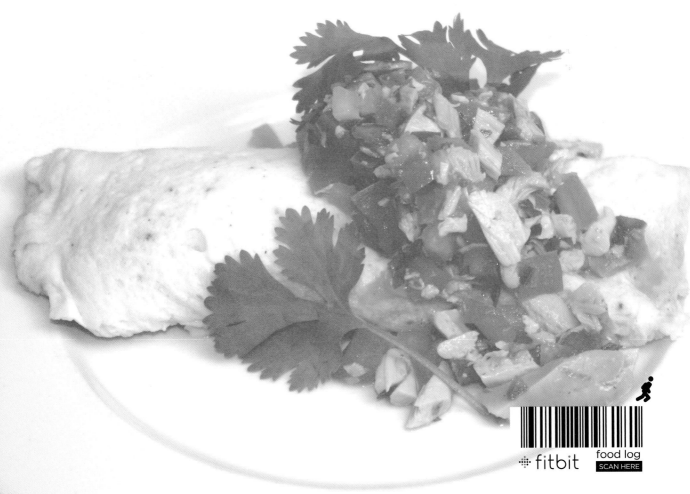

fitbit food log
SCAN HERE

BANANA SUPER YOGURT

THIS IS a great dish to take on the go because it literally improves as it sits! The chia seeds and underripe banana thicken the kefir to help you feel full during the day. Try adding my granola (page 116) in the jar, shake it once, and enjoy it right out of the jar. It's hard to compare to another food that is 99 percent lactose-free, has less than 2 grams of fat per serving, and is naturally sweetened, because there is none on the market!

Yield	Prep time	Processing time	Calorie Burn	Calories	Net-Calories
1 (5-ounce) serving	approximately 2 minutes	approximately 30 minutes	97	70	-27

Ingredients:

½   cup plain 99% lactose-free fat-free kefir (such as Lifeway)
1   teaspoon chia seeds
½   teaspoon psyllium husks (such as Yerba)
1½   teaspoons monk fruit crystals (such as Lakanto Golden Sweetener)
1   ounce slightly underripe banana

Method:

1. Place the kefir in a mason jar and add the chia seeds, psyllium, and monk fruit crystals. Chop the banana until mashed but stop before it starts to lose its body, about 1 minute.
2. Place the banana in the jar, seal tightly, and shake for at least 2 minutes. Refrigerate the jar for at least 30 minutes or up to 1 day. Remove the lid and enjoy.

Tip:

Try adding the CYBO granola right in the jar and shaking it once before consuming.

Per serving:

70 calories, 1.5g fat (0g sat), 2.5mg cholesterol, 60.5mg sodium, 21g carbohydrate, 3.1g fiber, 6.8g protein

Recommended Ready-Made Version:

Green Valley Lactose-free Vanilla Yogurt
Fat: 3g / Calories: 120 cal

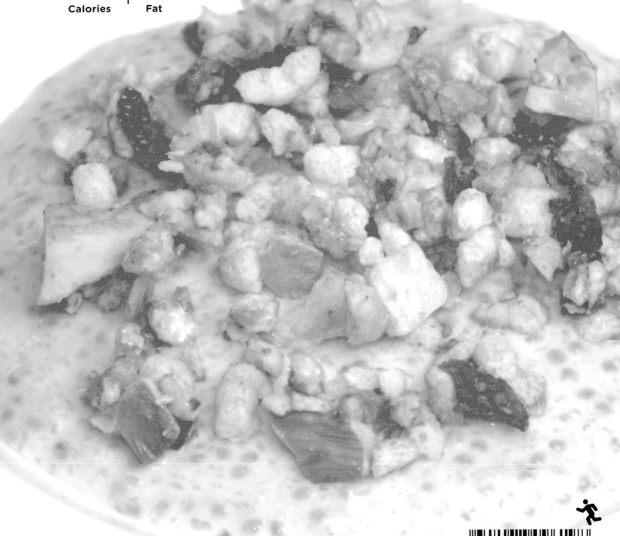

BEFORE

400 | **4**
Calories | Fat

AFTER

70 | **1.5**
Calories | Fat

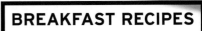

Shown with Fat-free, No-Sugar-Added Gluten-free Granola (see page 116)

FAT-FREE, NO-SUGAR-ADDED GLUTEN-FREE GRANOLA

GRANOLA, BY most standards, is an imposter. It goes by the name of "health food," but is anything but. Most granolas are loaded with sugar and fat—not exactly the combo you want for a slim, healthy body. Here's a granola that takes out the fat, the sugar, even the gluten, without sacrificing the delightful taste of traditional granola. Enjoy it with homemade 99 percent lactose-free Banana Super Yogurt (page 114), your favorite yogurt, or simply as a snack.

Yield	Prep time	Processing time	Calorie Burn	Calories	Net-Calories
½ cup	approximately 12 minutes	approximately 12 minutes	110	56.5	-53.5

Ingredients:

- Olive oil cooking spray
- ½ steamed chestnut
- 2 grams (about 2 tablespoons) gluten-free banana puffs (such as Happy Puffs; look near the baby food)
- ¼ unsalted brown rice cake (such as Lundberg; about 5 grams)
- 3.5 grams freeze-dried apple (such as Just Apples)
- 2 grams freeze-dried strawberries (such as Just Strawberries)
- ½ teaspoon coconut nectar (such as Coconut Secret)
- ½ packet monk fruit powder (such as Monk Fruit in the Raw)
- ½ packet stevia powder (such as Stevia in the Raw)
- Kosher salt

Method:

1. Preheat the oven to 325°F.
2. Spray a small nonstick ovenproof skillet with cooking spray and place it over medium-high heat. Lightly chop the chestnut into small pieces (but not so that it's powdery) and add it to the pan. Cook the chestnut, stirring, until it is beginning to toast. Transfer the pan to the oven and cook until the chestnut pieces are crisp, about 3 minutes. Leave the oven on.
3. Meanwhile, lightly chop the puffs, rice cake, and freeze-dried fruits into roughly ½-inch pieces. Remove the pan with the chestnut pieces from the oven and add the coconut nectar, monk fruit, stevia, and a pinch of salt. Add the chopped puffs and fruit and stir with a rubber spatula until everything is coated.
4. Scrape the mixture onto a nonstick baking sheet, spread it out in an even layer, and bake until dry and crisp, about 5 minutes. Stir the mixture after 5 minutes. Remove the pan from the oven and let cool.

Per serving:

56.5 calories, 0g fat (0g sat), 2.5mg cholesterol, 50mg sodium, 13.5g carbohydrate, 0.9g fiber, 0.45g protein

Recommended Ready-Made Version:

Purley Elizabeth ancient grain granola

Fat: 6g / Calories: 140 cal

BEFORE

226 | 0
Calories | Fat

AFTER

56.5 | 0
Calories | Fat

COOK YOUR BUTT OFF!

GREEN EGGS AND HAM

AS IN the Dr. Seuss book by the same name, I insist this dish is indeed a delectable meal to be savored at any breakfast. Enjoy!

Yield	Prep time	Processing time	Calorie Burn	Calories	Net-Calories
1 breakfast meal	approximately 10 minutes	approximately 10 minutes	100	103	3

Ingredients:

Olive oil cooking spray

1 **slice all-natural Canadian bacon (such as Applegate Farms)**

1 **tablespoon minced onions**

Red pepper flakes

2½ **ounces "triple-washed" spinach (¼ of a 10-ounce bag)**

Kosher salt

¼ **cup egg whites (such as Egg Beaters 100% Whites)**

1 **teaspoon egg white powder (such as Deb El Just Whites)**

Method:

1. Preheat the broiler. Spray a small nonstick ovenproof skillet with cooking spray, place it over medium-high heat, and add the Canadian bacon. Cook until browned on each side, about 20 seconds per side, then remove from the heat and set the bacon aside in a warm place.

2. Add the onions to the pan and reduce the heat to low. Cook the onions until softened, about 2 minutes. Add a pinch of red pepper flakes, then the spinach, and raise the heat to medium-high. Cook the spinach until it is wilted and soft and all the water has evaporated from it, about 3 minutes. Season with salt and place the spinach and onion mixture on a cutting board. Chop the mixture until it is pulverized to the point of a puree.

3. In a small bowl, whisk together the egg whites and egg white powder until they have formed soft peaks. Add the spinach mixture and season lightly with salt. Return the mixture to the skillet and cook over medium-high heat until the eggs have just about set, then spread the eggs into an even layer and place under the broiler until they are cooked through and the water has evaporated, about 30 seconds.

4. Slide the eggs onto a plate, add the Canadian bacon, and serve.

Per serving:

103 calories, 2g fat (0.8g sat), 17.5mg cholesterol, 431.25mg sodium, 5.5g carbohydrate, 1.7g fiber, 16.29g protein

Recommended Ready-Made Version:

Cedarlane Spinach and Mushroom Egg White Omelette
Fat: 12g / Calories: 270 cal

BEFORE

665 | 51
Calories | Fat

AFTER

103 | 2
Calories | Fat

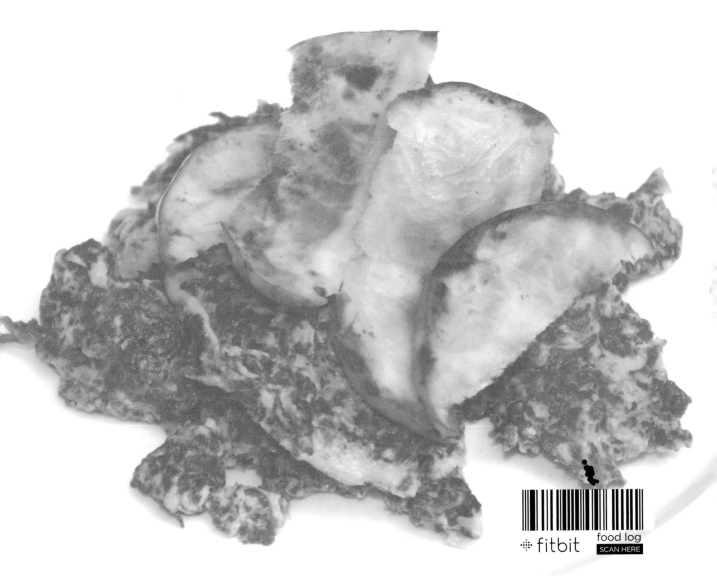

fitbit food log
SCAN HERE

COOK YOUR BUTT OFF!

CHAPTER 8

Lunch Recipes

Wrap with Shrimp and Tomato Salad

*Ham and Tomato Panini
with Spicy Mayo*

Turkey and Avocado Sandwich

Vegetarian Chili Burger

Crispy Taco Shells and Bean Chili

Open-faced Mushroom Salad

Pulled-Pork Sandwich

Brussels Sprouts with Chicken

*Chopped Shiitake and Noodle Salad
with Bok Choy*

WRAP WITH SHRIMP AND TOMATO SALAD

WRAPS ARE the new sandwiches. But there are a lot of nutritional bad guys wrapped up in them: gluten, fat, calories, and carbs, to name just a few. My rendition exiles the bad guys, so you can enjoy it guilt free. The wrap alone has about 3g of carbs and is only 41 calories for a 9-inch wrap! In fact, this entire dish contains fewer calories than you'll find in any wrap.

Yield	Prep time	Processing time	Calorie Burn	Calories	Net-Calories
1 wrap	approximately 20 minutes	approximately 5 minutes	56	177	121

Ingredients:

6	tablespoons cold water
2	teaspoons psyllium husk flakes
1	tablespoon plus 2 teaspoons egg white powder (such as Deb El Just Whites)
	Kosher salt and freshly ground black pepper
	Olive oil cooking spray
¾	cup shredded green cabbage
2	ounces peeled cooked shrimp, halved lengthwise
5	tablespoons prepared pico de gallo (such as Ready Pac)
¼	cup fresh cilantro, lightly chopped
¼	ripe avocado, diced
	Zest and juice of ½ lime
½	lime, for serving

Method:

1. Preheat the oven to 350°F.
2. Pour the water into a large bowl, add the psyllium, and whisk until all the psyllium has dissolved and the water is slightly thickened, about 2 minutes. Add the egg white powder, season with salt and pepper, and whisk slowly to dissolve the egg white but not aerate it, about 1 minute.
3. Spray a 12-inch nonstick ovenproof skillet with cooking spray and pour the egg white mixture into the skillet. Tilt the pan so the mixture covers the bottom of the pan completely. Place over medium-high heat and cook until the bottom is beginning to solidify, about 30 seconds. Place the pan in the oven and bake until the top is cooked, about 30 seconds. Place the pan back on the stovetop over medium-high heat, flip to lightly brown the other side, then slide off onto a plate and set aside.
4. Chop the cabbage and shrimp into small pieces and place both in a bowl. Add the pico de gallo and cilantro and season with salt and pepper. Add the avocado, lime zest, and juice to the bowl and mix. Evenly spoon the mixture onto the wrap. Fold the wrap and serve with the other half of the lime.

Tip:

Add some jalapeños or hot sauce to spice things up a bit for about 1 calorie more per serving.

Per serving:

177 calories, 6g fat (.4g sat, 0g mono, 0g poly), 110.5mg cholesterol, 299mg sodium, 13g carbohydrate, 6.75g fiber, 21g protein

Recommended Ready-Made Version:

Amy's Gluten Free Non Dairy Burrito
Fat: 6g / Calories: 240 cal

BEFORE

640 | 22
Calories | Fat

AFTER

177 | 6
Calories | Fat

fitbit food log
SCAN HERE

HAM AND TOMATO PANINI WITH SPICY MAYO

YOU'LL BE hooked on this hot and crispy panini—a new twist on the classic comfort-food ham and cheese sandwich. I've chosen uncured ham here—free of preservatives and other nasty additives. This panini is made with a gluten-free dough, too, and the results are amazing.

Yield	Prep time	Processing time	Calorie Burn	Calories	Net-Calories
1 sandwich	approximately 5 minutes	approximately 10 minutes	112	215.5	103.5

Ingredients:

52	grams (about 1¾ ounces) gluten-free pizza dough (such as Gillian's)
½	red jalapeño
2¼	teaspoons light canola mayonnaise (such as Spectrum)
¼	teaspoon white wine vinegar
2	ounces uncured smoked ham (such as Applegate Farms)
1	large leaf romaine lettuce
2	slices ripe tomato, each about ½ inch thick
	Kosher salt

Method:

1. Place a cast-iron griddle (the flat side of a stovetop griddle) or cast-iron pan over medium-high heat. Place the pizza dough between two pieces of plastic wrap and roll it into a rectangular shape about ⅛ inch thick.
2. Cook the dough on the griddle on both sides until cooked and crisp, about 1 minute per side. Transfer to a cutting board and cut each flatbread in half crosswise.
3. Mince the jalapeño into a fine paste and mix with the mayo and vinegar in a small bowl.
4. Assemble the sandwich by evenly spreading the spicy mayo on one side of the flatbread pieces, then top one flatbread with the ham, lettuce, and tomato slices. Season the tomato slices with salt and place the remaining piece of flatbread on top to close the sandwiches. Place the finished sandwich on the griddle once more to warm the sandwich while gently pressing. Cut the sandwich in half and serve.

Tips:

- Use only 1 ounce of ham and save 25 calories!
- Add 4 torn basil leaves for a fresh addition and next to no calories.

Per serving:

215.5 calories, 7g fat (0.5g sat), 35mg cholesterol, 674mg sodium, 26.1g carbohydrate, 1.25g fiber, 14g protein

Recommended Ready-Made Version:

Gluten-free Pocket Sandwich Ham and Cheddar
Fat: 15g / Calories: 270 cal

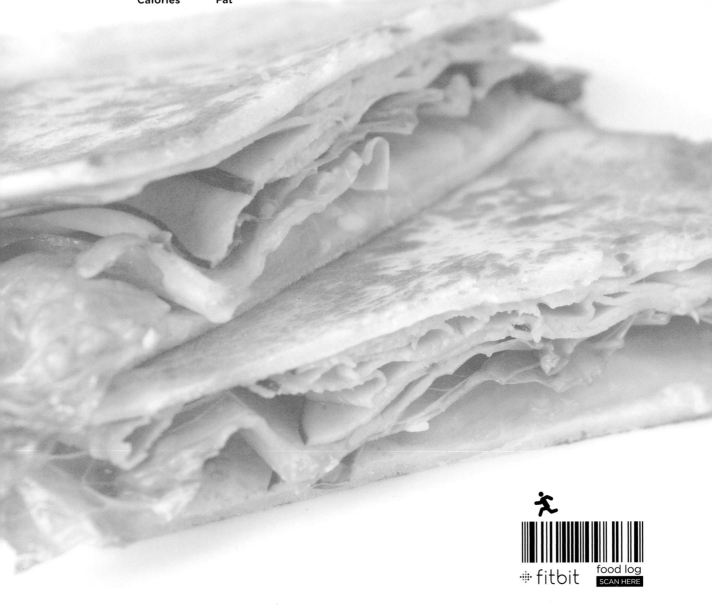

BEFORE

801 | 50
Calories | Fat

AFTER

215.5 | 7
Calories | Fat

fitbit
food log
SCAN HERE

TURKEY AND AVOCADO SANDWICH

HERE'S ANOTHER panini (yes, I am hooked on them), one that features a high-health ingredient: avocado. This creamy fruit is filled with good fats, vitamins, minerals, and fiber. Avocado fills in for mayo anytime, and I love it on just about any sandwich, wrap, or panini.

Yield	Prep time	Processing time	Calorie Burn	Calories	Net-Calories
1 sandwich	approximately 5 minutes	approximately 15 minutes	89	279	190

Ingredients:

52	grams (about 1¾ ounces) gluten-free pizza dough (such as Gillian's)
¼	ripe Hass avocado, peeled and mashed
2	ounces store-roasted turkey, thinly sliced
¾	cup radish or alfalfa sprouts, or your favorite!
¼	cup very thin slices unpeeled Granny Smith apple
1	teaspoon Dijon mustard

Method:

1. Place a cast-iron griddle (the flat side of a stovetop griddle) or cast-iron pan over medium-high heat. Place the pizza dough between two pieces of plastic wrap and using a rolling pin, roll into a rectangular shape about ⅛ inch thick.
2. Cook the dough on the griddle on both sides until cooked and crisp, about 1 minute per side. Transfer to a cutting board and cut the flatbread in half crosswise.
3. Assemble the sandwich by evenly spreading the avocado on one side of each of the flatbread pieces, then top one piece of flatbread with the turkey, the sprouts, and finally the apple. Spread the mustard on the remaining piece of flatbread and place the remaining piece of flatbread on top to close the sandwich. Place the finished sandwich on the griddle once more to warm the sandwich while gently pressing. Cut the sandwich in half and serve.

Per serving:

279 calories, 9g fat (0.85g sat), 47mg cholesterol, 410mg sodium, 29g carbohydrate, 2.95g fiber, 21g protein

Recommended Ready-Made Version:

Unfortunately, there are no readily available gluten-free, low calorie sandwich solutions. Looks like you will just have to make mine!

BEFORE

950 | 64
Calories | **Fat**

AFTER

279 | 9
Calories | **Fat**

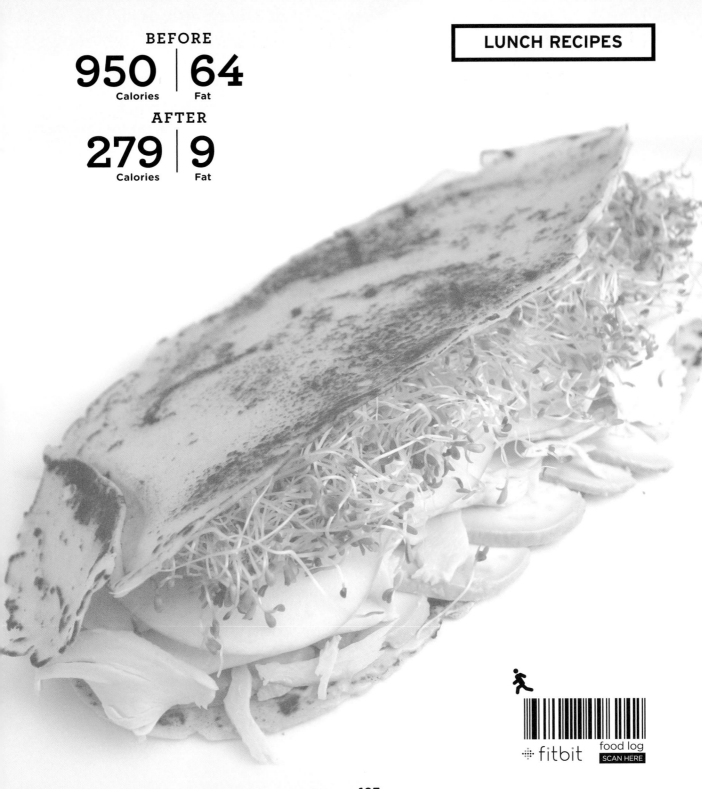

fitbit food log
SCAN HERE

127

VEGETARIAN CHILI BURGER

EVERY MEATLESS "burger" I've ever tried has fallen short of desirable, so I tried to create one that I could really sink my teeth into—plus help people who want to follow a more plant-based diet. I spent a lot of time coming up with this recipe, and I must say, I love, *love* this burger! It looks like a burger, it feels like a burger, it contains no meat, and it can be made in no time flat. Egg white powder holds everything together. The centerpiece here is the cremini mushroom, which has a naturally meaty taste (as do the black beans). And I just love that these tasty mushrooms are bun-sized.

Yield	Prep time	Processing time	Calorie Burn	Calories	Net-Calories
1 veggie burger	approximately 15 minutes	approximately 10 minutes	110	80	-30

Ingredients:

2   tablespoons drained no-salt-added black beans (such as Eden)
3   ounces cremini mushrooms, gills removed with a spoon
1¾ ounces peeled grated raw beet (about ⅓ cup)
    Kosher salt and freshly ground black pepper
    Chili powder
2½ teaspoons egg white powder (such as Deb El Just Whites)
    Olive oil cooking spray

Method:

1. Preheat the oven to 350°F.
2. Place the black beans in a mortar and use the pestle to mash them, then scrape the mashed beans into a bowl. Chop the mushrooms until they are almost a puree. Add the mushrooms and beets to the bowl with the black beans and mix well with a spoon until you have a loose paste. Season with salt, pepper, and chili powder and add the egg white powder. Mix well with a spoon until smooth.
3. Form the mixture into a patty about ¾ inch thick on a parchment paper square. Spray a large nonstick ovenproof skillet with cooking spray and place it over medium-high heat. Once the pan is hot, gently slide the patty into the pan. Cook the patty until the bottom is browned and it has started to firm up, 2 to 3 minutes. Spray the top of the patty with cooking spray, flip, and cook until the other side is beginning to brown. Place the pan in the oven and cook until the patty is firm, 2 to 3 minutes.
4. Remove the pan from the oven and place the cooked patty on a plate. Serve as desired (see Tips, below).

Tips:

• Use only the freshest mushrooms for this recipe or the burger's flavor could be compromised.
• I like to put this burger between two large romaine leaves and eat it with my hands for a quick lunch.
• Serve on my Gluten-free Roll (p. 212) with 2 tablespoons stevia-sweetened ketchup for a great burger and 190 cals!
• These can be cooked ahead of time and just reheated in a toaster oven.
• Add ¼ of an avocado, mashed up, for an additional 57 calories and 5g of fat.

- If you can tolerate a little lactose, try topping the patty with 1 ounce of grated 75 percent reduced-fat cheddar cheese (such as Cabot) for an additional 60 calories and 2.5g of fat.

Per serving:

80 calories, 0.5g fat (0.05g sat), 0mg cholesterol, 741 mg sodium, 15.55g carbohydrate, 4g fiber, 8.1g protein

Recommended Ready-Made Version:

Boca Cheeseburger
Fat: 4.5g / Calories: 100 cal

BEFORE

270 | **18**
Calories | Fat

AFTER

80 | **0.5**
Calories | Fat

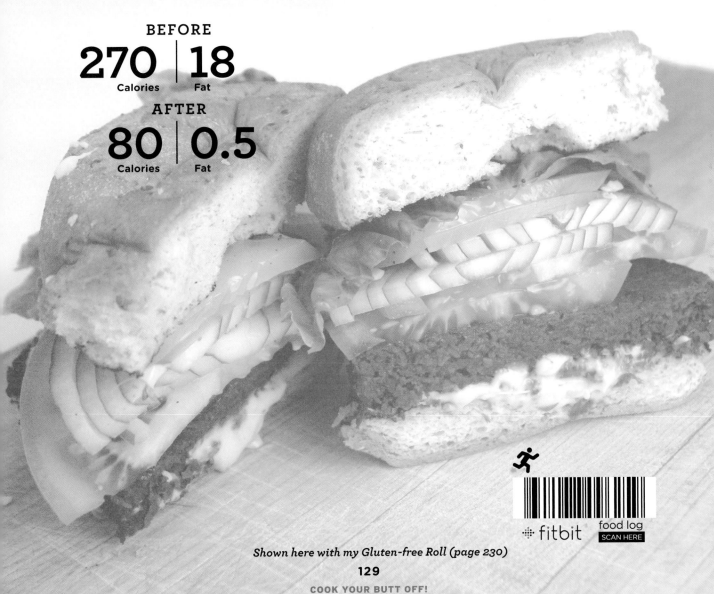

Shown here with my Gluten-free Roll (page 230)

CRISPY TACO SHELLS AND BEAN CHILI

DON'T BE afraid to make your own taco shells for this dish. Before you run for the border, it's simply a matter of mixing psyllium husk powder, arrowroot powder, and egg white powder, patting the mixture into flat rounds, and baking them in the oven. These homemade tacos have all the savory depth you expect from the store-bought variety and virtually no carbs. The real prize, though, is the chili filling.

Yield	Prep time	Processing time	Calorie Burn	Calories	Net-Calories
1 taco	approximately 10 minutes	approximately 20 minutes	132	172.5	40.5

Ingredients:

- 2 tablespoons water
- 2 tablespoons psyllium husk powder (such as Yerba)
- ½ teaspoon arrowroot powder
- 2 teaspoons egg white powder (such as Deb El Just Whites)
- Kosher salt and freshly ground black pepper
- ½ cup reduced-sodium Southwestern bean chili (such as Amy's)
- ½ cup shredded iceberg lettuce
- 2 tablespoons plain fat-free Greek yogurt (such as Fage 0%)
- ¼ cup fresh cilantro sprigs
- ¼ lime, cut into wedges

Method:

1. Preheat the oven to 325°F.
2. In a small bowl, whisk together the psyllium and arrowroot with the water until thick, then add the egg white powder and mix until smooth. Season with salt and pepper. Roll the mixture between oven-safe waxed paper into a rounded rectangle about ⅛ inch thick and about 6 inches long and 4 inches wide. Place on a baking sheet and bake until it is cooked through but still floppy, about 5 minutes.
3. Place the cooked dough over the side of a microwave-safe straight-sided coffee mug and microwave on high until beginning to crisp but still pliable, about 1 minute. Fold the shell in half like a taco shell and tuck it inside the mug so it keeps its shape. Microwave until very crisp, about 1 minute. Remove and set aside.
4. Pour the chili into a microwave-safe bowl and microwave on high until hot, about 2 minutes. Place the lettuce on the taco shell, followed by the chili. Dollop with yogurt, top with cilantro, and serve with lime wedges.

Tip:

This shell recipe also makes amazing tortilla chips. Simply cut into triangle shapes and cook flat until crisp and have a snack of tortilla chips for only 40 calories and 1 net carb!

Per serving:

172.5 calories, 2g fat (0.25g sat), 0mg cholesterol, 383mg sodium, 31.7g carbohydrate, 12g fiber, 6.3g protein

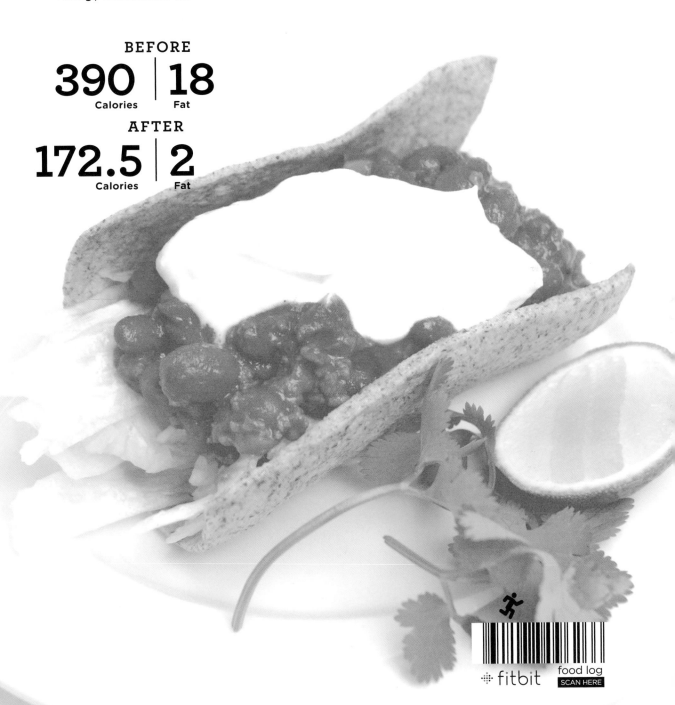

Recommended Ready-Made Version:

Amy's bean-and-rice non-dairy burrito
Fat: 8g / Calories: 320 cal

BEFORE

390 | 18
Calories | Fat

AFTER

172.5 | 2
Calories | Fat

fitbit food log SCAN HERE

OPEN-FACED MUSHROOM SALAD

MUSHROOMS are valued not only for their savory, meaty taste, but also for their medicinal value in boosting immunity. This salad is warm—and thus delicious in cool weather. The warm temperature of the mushroom activates the release of the natural fat in the olives. The result is a taste sensation that feels lusciously high fat, although the salad is super lean.

Yield	Prep time	Processing time	Calorie Burn	Calories	Net-Calories
1 large salad	approximately 5 minutes	approximately 20 minutes	47	99.25	52.25

Ingredients:

1	(4-ounce) stemless portabello mushroom
	Kosher salt and freshly ground black pepper
1	cup chopped romaine hearts
¼	cup bottled roasted red peppers, cut into bite-sized pieces
2	pieces bottled water-packed artichoke hearts (such as Progresso), drained
½	ounce pitted ripe black olives, chopped (about 3 tablespoons)
4	fresh basil leaves
1	teaspoon hot cherry pepper brine

Method:

1. Scrape the gills from the mushroom. Place the mushroom on a microwave-safe plate, gill-side up, and season with salt and pepper. Microwave on high until the mushroom starts to steam and become tender, about 2 minutes. Flip the mushroom and microwave on high until cooked, 1 to 2 minutes more. Transfer to a plate and set aside.
2. Place the remaining ingredients in a bowl, season lightly with salt and pepper, and toss to mix well. Spoon the lettuce mixture into the mushroom and serve.

Tip:

Add 1 cup of no-salt-added chickpeas to the lettuce mixture for a little added protein and creamy texture for an additional 67 calories per serving.

Per serving:

99.25 calories, 2.45g fat (1.975g sat, 0g mono, 0g poly), 0mg cholesterol, 555mg sodium, 17.6g carbohydrate, 5.75g fiber, 4g protein

Recommended Ready-Made Version:

Chop't Salad with Lite Balsamic dressing
Fat: 3g / Calories: 85 cal

BEFORE

396.2 | 35.9
Calories | Fat

AFTER

99.25 | 2.5
Calories | Fat

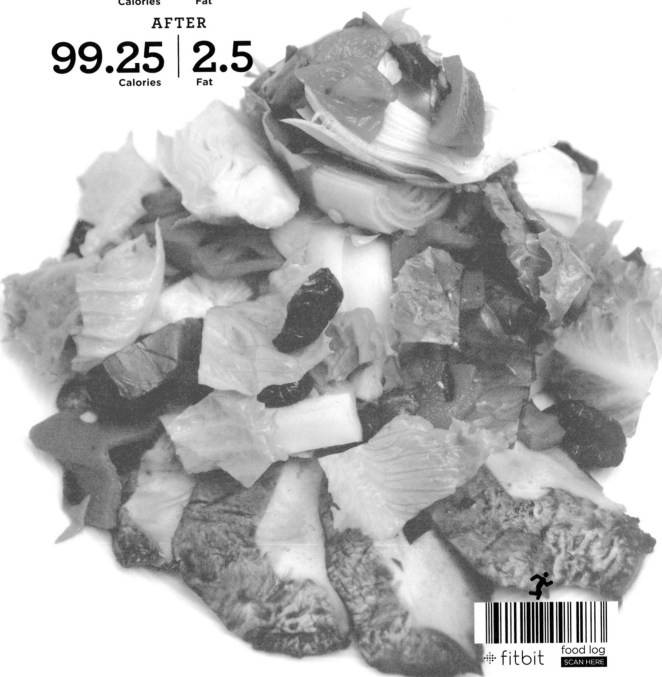

fitbit food log
SCAN HERE

PULLED-PORK SANDWICH

I CRAVE good old-fashioned barbecue just about any time of the year. My favorite is a tender pulled-pork sandwich—that moist, flavorful meat simmered in a thick sauce and nestled in a big bun. My version of this sandwich, however, demonstrates most of the techniques I use to skinny-up the fattening foods we love to eat—techniques that took me years to perfect. Starting with precooked lean pork loin, I add sugar-free ketchup, red wine vinegar, and liquid smoke for pure barbecue flavor in a dish with slashed calories. I love the fact that I can buy so many gluten-free breads now, and that's what I've used here.

Yield	Prep time	Processing time	Calorie Burn	Calories	Net-Calories
1 open-faced sandwich	approximately 5 minutes	approximately 20 minutes	52	197	145

Ingredients:

2   tablespoons no-sugar-added ketchup (such as AlternaSweets)
2¼   teaspoons red wine vinegar
½   tablespoon liquid smoke
3   ounces cooked pork loin, fat trimmed, thinly sliced by your deli
     Kosher salt and freshly ground black pepper
1   slice gluten-free whole-grain bread (such as Udi's), halved

Method:

1. Preheat the broiler.
2. In a microwave-safe bowl, mix together the ketchup, vinegar, and liquid smoke. Place the pork on a cutting board and chop into tiny pieces. Add the pork to the bowl with the ketchup mixture, season with salt and pepper, cover with parchment paper, and microwave until hot, about 2 minutes.
3. Place the bread slice on a baking sheet and toast cut-side up under the broiler.
4. Evenly distribute the pork on the toasted bread slice and serve open-faced.

Tips:

• Add 1 leaf of butter lettuce to each sandwich for an extra calorie per serving.
• Add some jalapeños or hot sauce to spice things up a bit for about 1 calorie more per serving.
• Add 1 packet of monk fruit powder to the ketchup if you like a sweeter BBQ sauce.

Per serving:

197 calories, 3g fat (1g sat, 0g mono, 0g poly), 62mg cholesterol, 540mg sodium, 13g carbohydrate, 1g fiber, 31.5g protein

Recommended Ready-Made Version:

O' Tasty Foods
Fat: 13g / Calories: 360 cal

BEFORE

862 | **45**
Calories | Fat

AFTER

197 | **3**
Calories | Fat

fitbit food log SCAN HERE

COOK YOUR BUTT OFF!

BRUSSELS SPROUTS WITH CHICKEN

I LOVE A good pasta dish with Brussels sprouts. I wanted to re-create that dish, but before I added the pasta, I took a taste. The mashed Brussels sprouts tasted so good that they needed no pasta. I cut a little leftover chicken breast into pieces about the size of rigatoni and tossed it in, thus saving on carbs and calories and boosting the protein content of the dish. I recommend adding grated Parmigiano-Reggiano (or even Pecorino Romano) if you can afford the extra 28 calories. You know what I love most about this dish? It tastes as good cold as it does hot—so pack it up to go!

Yield	Prep time	Processing time	Calorie Burn	Calories	Net-Calories
1 lunch meal	approximately 15 minutes	approximately 15 minutes	157	147	-10

Ingredients:

Olive oil cooking spray

6 **large Brussels sprouts, trimmed**

Kosher salt

1 **teaspoon minced garlic**

Pinch of red pepper flakes

¼ **cup chopped fresh parsley**

Scant sprinkle of ground cinnamon

⅛ **teaspoon paprika**

½ **cup chicken stock**

2½ **ounces cooked boneless skinless chicken breast, sliced**

¼ **ounce grated Parmigiano-Reggiano (about 7 grams; optional)**

Method:

1. Preheat the oven to 400°F.
2. Spray a large nonstick ovenproof pan with cooking spray and place it over medium-high heat. Cut the Brussels sprouts in half from top to stem and place them cut-side down in the pan. Cook until the edges begin to brown, then season with salt and place in the oven to roast until tender, about 8 minutes.
3. Remove the sprouts from the pan and set aside. Add the garlic to the pan and cook, stirring, until golden brown, about 30 seconds. Add the red pepper flakes to the pan, then add the parsley and cook until wilted. Add the spices and the stock and bring to a simmer.
4. Chop the Brussels sprouts on a cutting board until they're mostly mashed but with some bite-sized pieces and add to the pan. Add the chicken breast and cook until the stock and Brussels sprouts stick to the chicken as if it were pasta. Spoon the mixture into a bowl and top with the Parmigiano-Reggiano, if desired.

Per serving:

147 calories, 1.5g fat (0.3g sat), 41mg cholesterol, 168.5mg sodium, 12.5g carbohydrate, 5g fiber, 23.35g protein

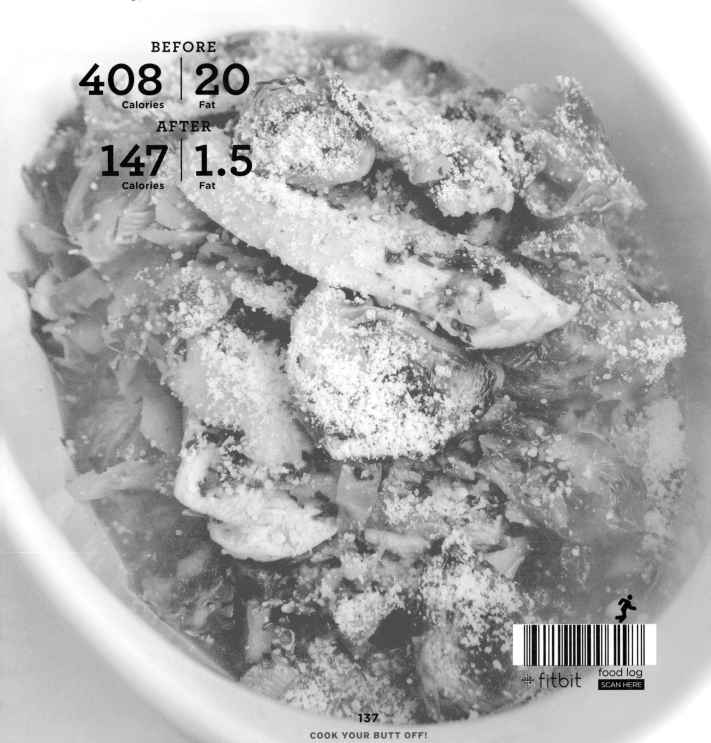

Recommended Ready-Made Version:

Lean Cuisine Glazed Chicken
Fat: 5g / Calories: 240 cal

BEFORE
408 | **20**
Calories | Fat

AFTER
147 | **1.5**
Calories | Fat

fitbit food log
SCAN HERE

CHOPPED SHIITAKE AND NOODLE SALAD WITH BOK CHOY

HERE'S A great dish to take on the road. The dried mushroom flavor just grows as it sits and really grounds the exotic flavor of the salad. Those mushrooms do more than just taste delicious; they're also healing and known to strengthen the immune system.

Yield	Prep time	Processing time	Calorie Burn	Calories	Net-Calories
1 salad	approximately 15 minutes	approximately 15 minutes	167	87	-80

Ingredients:

1 tablespoon gluten-free reduced-sodium tamari (such as San-J)
1 teaspoon chopped jalapeño
1 teaspoon white wine vinegar
1 dried shiitake mushroom
2 bags shirataki spaghetti (such as Miracle Noodle)
4 whole shiitake mushrooms, stems removed
1 cup chopped baby bok choy
⅛ teaspoon grated orange zest
2½ tablespoons orange segments, cut into small chunks, with any juice they release
¼ cup roughly chopped fresh cilantro

Method:

1. In a small bowl, combine the tamari, jalapeño, and vinegar, and, using a Microplane, grate the dried shiitake into the tamari mixture. Cover and let stand at room temperature.

2. Place the noodles in a large salad spinner. Rinse under cold water until they smell fresh and then spin in the salad spinner to dry. Transfer the noodles to a cutting board and chop them into small bite-sized pieces.

3. Place a nonstick skillet over medium-high heat and add the chopped noodles to the pan. Cook until they have evaporated all of their water and place in a bowl.

4. Roughly chop the fresh shiitakes, add half of them to the pan, and cook until they begin to release some water. Transfer the cooked mushrooms to the bowl with the noodles and add the remaining mushrooms. Add the bok choy, orange zest, and orange pieces and any juice they released to the tamari mixture and pour it over the salad. Toss to coat. Add the cilantro, toss, check the seasoning and spoon onto a plate to serve.

Tips:

• Try omitting the noodles and adding ½ cup of cooked brown rice for an added 115 calories and 1g of fat.
• Add 2 ounces of cooked lean protein to this dish for about 50 calories more.

Per serving:

87 calories, 0.5g fat (0.15g sat), 0mg cholesterol, 774mg sodium, 16g carbohydrate, 4.75g fiber, 6.4g protein

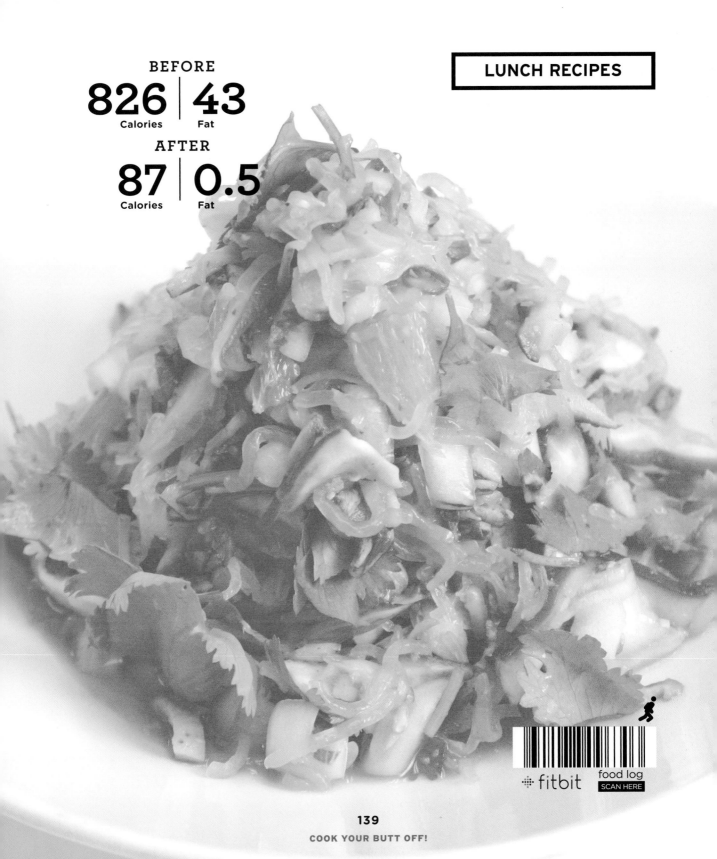

BEFORE

826 | **43**
Calories | Fat

AFTER

87 | **0.5**
Calories | Fat

fitbit | food log
SCAN HERE

Chicken with Glazed Eggplant and
Cauliflower Rice

Chicken and Mushrooms Balsamico

Chicken Teriyaki with Fresh Sugar
Snap Peas

Chicken with Artichokes and Rosemary

Chicken with Marinated Bean Sprouts

Chicken with Parsley, Peppers, and
Lemon

Chili-rubbed Chicken with Black Bean
Salsa and Rice

Cod with Tomatoes, Zucchini,
and Black Olives

Meat Loaf with Mashed Sweet Potatoes

CHAPTER 9

Dinner Recipes

Pumpkin Risotto with Sage

Asian Pork Buns

Roasted Pork with Sauerkraut, Apples, and Dijon Mustard

Grilled Hearts of Romaine with Marinated Shrimp

Soy Spaghetti with Shrimp and Hand-chopped Pomodoro Sauce

Spaghetti with Asparagus Pesto and Pecorino Romano

Spinach Dumplings with Marinara

Sweet Potato Spaetzle

Vegetable Fried "Rice"

CHICKEN WITH GLAZED EGGPLANT AND CAULIFLOWER RICE

SKINLESS CHICKEN has become sort of like cottage cheese, the ubiquitous base upon which many weight-loss diets are built. But it doesn't register well on the ol' excitement meter. I mean, how many times have you found yourself craving a naked, unseasoned piece of chicken? Not me—I'd throw up the white flag and order pizza if the road to lasting weight loss looked like an endless parade of plain chicken breasts.

Take the advice of a guy who has gobbled up his fair share of chicken: Don't abandon it altogether, but do what you can to break up the monotony. Especially during dieting, it's important not to get lazy in your chicken prep, and it's just as important to add some perk to your poultry. That's why I prefer to use chicken thighs over breasts, like I do in this recipe. Thighs are meatier and more flavorful, but still low in calories.

Yield	Prep time	Processing time	Calorie Burn	Calories	Net-Calories
1 main course	**approximately 15 minutes**	**approximately 15 minutes**	**157**	**190**	**33**

Ingredients:

Olive oil cooking spray

3 **tablespoons grated cauliflower (grated on the large side of a box grater)**

Kosher salt and red pepper flakes

1 **(4-ounce) boneless skinless chicken thigh (or breast if you insist), scored crosswise ¼ inch deep**

1½ **cups eggplant, cut into 2-inch pieces**

1 **large clove garlic, thinly sliced**

1 **teaspoon chopped peeled fresh ginger**

1 **tablespoon gluten-free reduced-sodium tamari (such as San-J)**

½ **tablespoon balsamic vinegar**

Method:

1. Spray a large nonstick pan with cooking spray and place it over medium-high heat. Add the grated cauliflower and cook, stirring, until it is softened and just tender, about 1 minute. Season with salt and red pepper flakes, spoon onto a plate, and set aside.

2. Wipe the pan dry then spray again with cooking spray and place it over medium-high heat. Season the chicken with salt and cook until browned and cooked through, about 2 minutes. Transfer to a plate and set aside. Add the eggplant to the pan and cook until browned and soft, about 5 minutes, then move the eggplant to the side of the pan, add the garlic, and cook until browned, about 30 seconds. Add the ginger and cook until aromatic, about 15 seconds more.

3. Add the tamari and vinegar to the pan along with a splash of water and return the chicken to the pan. Cook until the chicken is cooked through and the sauce sticks to everything, about 30 seconds. Place the chicken over the cauliflower rice and spoon the eggplant alongside. Serve with red pepper flakes.

Tips:

- Serve with a wedge of fresh lime and ¼ cup of fresh cilantro leaves for a burst of freshness for an additional 4 calories.
- If you like a sweeter sauce, try adding ½ tablespoon raw agave nectar for an additional 30 calories.

Per serving:

190 calories, 2g fat (1g sat), 70mg cholesterol, 823mg sodium, 16.06g carbohydrate, 5.4g fiber, 30.15g protein

Recommended Ready-Made Version:

Lean Cuisine Glazed Chicken
Fat: 5g / Calories: 240 cal

BEFORE

1,240 | **25**
Calories | Fat

AFTER

190 | **2**
Calories | Fat

fitbit food log SCAN HERE

CHICKEN AND MUSHROOMS BALSAMICO

A GREAT way to cut back on animal meat in certain recipes is to use mushrooms. Why mushrooms? They actually have a meaty flavor all their own—and trust me, no one will ever know that this recipe has less poultry in it for that reason. Plus, using mushrooms as a meat substitute cuts way back on calories and fat. The chunks of iceberg on top give a nice fresh quality to this dish—and will keep you full and satisfied.

Yield	Prep time	Processing time	Calorie Burn	Calories	Net-Calories
1 main course	approximately 15 minutes	approximately 15 minutes	102	152	50

Ingredients:

Olive oil cooking spray

3 ounces boneless skinless chicken thighs, cut into large chunks

Kosher salt and freshly ground black pepper

1 teaspoon chopped fresh rosemary

4 ounces whole cremini or baby bella mushrooms, sliced

¼ cup chopped onion

2 tablespoons balsamic vinegar

¼ chunk iceberg lettuce, cut into 3-inch chunks (about 1½ cups)

Method:

1. Spray a nonstick skillet with cooking spray and place it over medium-high heat. Season the chicken with salt and pepper and cook until brown on one side, about 2 minutes. Flip the chicken and brown the other side, about 1 minute, then add the rosemary and cook for 20 seconds. Transfer the chicken to a plate and set aside.
2. Spray the pan again with cooking spray, add the mushrooms, and allow them to brown, about 3 minutes. Transfer the mushrooms to a plate and set aside. Add the onions to the pan and cook until softened, about 2 minutes. Return the chicken and mushrooms to the pan, add the vinegar, and cook until the chicken is cooked through and the mixture has reduced to a saucelike consistency, about 3 minutes.
3. Season with salt and pepper and spoon the mixture evenly onto a plate. Spread the iceberg on top, scrape any of the pan sauce out over the lettuce, and serve.

Per serving:

152 calories, 3g fat (0.75g sat), 63.75mg cholesterol, 213.25mg sodium, 14g carbohydrate, 2.2g fiber, 19g protein

Recommended Ready-Made Version:

Lean Cuisine Glazed Chicken

Fat: 7.1g / Calories: 330 cal

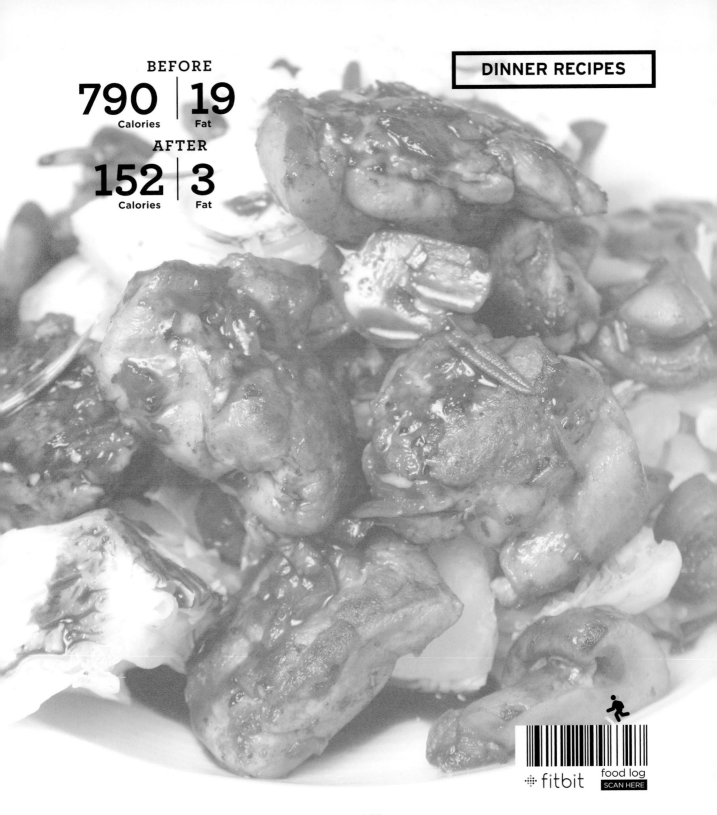

BEFORE

790
Calories

19
Fat

AFTER

152
Calories

3
Fat

fitbit food log
SCAN HERE

CHICKEN TERIYAKI WITH FRESH SUGAR SNAP PEAS

OVER THE years, this Japanese entrée has been the centerpiece on most Asian menus. While delicious, it's usually about chicken candied in sugar and soy and served with copious amounts of white rice. This is not a recipe for good health! Here is a much easier interpretation—with fewer calories, fat, and sodium and less sugar. Healthful doesn't mean tasteless! This recipe tastes delicious, even though I swapped out several fattening ingredients. For example, I replaced the sugary sauce with a sugar-free version of teriyaki sauce and traded in the rice for snap peas. Voilà—Chicken Teriyaki can now be declared a health food!

Yield	Prep time	Processing time	Calorie Burn	Calories	Net-Calories
1 main course	approximately 10 minutes	approximately 10 minutes	125	199	74

Ingredients:

Kosher salt

1 heaping cup trimmed fresh sugar snap peas

¾ teaspoon wasabi powder (such as Eden), mixed with 1 tablespoon water

1 ounce lite soft tofu (such as Nasoya), drained and diced

Olive oil cooking spray

1 (4-ounce) boneless skinless chicken cutlet

Freshly ground black pepper

2¼ teaspoons gluten-free reduced-sodium tamari (such as San-J)

2 teaspoons grated fresh okra (grated on a Microplane)

⅛ teaspoon grated lemon zest

¼ teaspoon fresh lemon juice

2 teaspoons monk fruit crystals (such as Lakanto Golden Sweetener)

½ packet stevia powder (such as Stevia in the Raw)

Method:

1. Pour 2 quarts of water into a wide saucepan, add a pinch of salt, and bring to a simmer over high heat. Add the peas and cook until bright green but still snappy, about 30 seconds. Drain and place in a bowl with the wasabi. Season with salt and add the tofu.

2. Meanwhile, spray a large nonstick skillet with cooking spray and place it over medium-high heat. Season the chicken with salt and pepper and cook until browned on both sides, about 1 minute per side. Remove from the heat.

3. Place the tamari, okra, lemon zest, lemon juice, monk fruit crystals, and stevia in a mason jar, seal the lid tightly, and shake vigorously until the mixture is thick, about 1 minute. Pour the mixture over the chicken, place over medium-high heat, and toss to coat the chicken until the sauce is hot and sticks to the chicken.

4. Place the chicken on a plate and place the pea mixture into the pan and warm in the remaining sauce. Spoon the pea mixture next to the chicken and serve.

Tip:

Add 1 tablespoon of chopped scallions for only 2 extra calories.

Per serving:

199 calories, 2g fat (0.4g sat), 65.75mg cholesterol, 620mg sodium, 17.3g carbohydrate, 3.15g fiber, 33g protein

Recommended Ready-Made Version:

Lean Cuisine Chicken Teriyaki Stir Fry
Fat: 2g / Calories: 250 cal

BEFORE
430 | 7
Calories | Fat

AFTER
199 | 2
Calories | Fat

fitbit food log
SCAN HERE

COOK YOUR BUTT OFF!

CHICKEN WITH ARTICHOKES AND ROSEMARY

THIS RECIPE screams good-for-you! Garlic is good for your heart and immune system. Artichokes are liver detoxifiers, plus high in fiber for bowel health. And rosemary—well, it's a brain and memory booster. All three complement chicken cutlets, which are super low in fat and loaded with protein. Did I mention that this dish tastes good, too? You can eat and enjoy this recipe, guilt free, and feel like you're eating something that's fancy-schmancy, elegant, and infinitely good for your health.

Yield	Prep time	Processing time	Calorie Burn	Calories	Net-Calories
1 main course	**approximately 15 minutes**	**approximately 15 minutes**	**149**	**176**	**27**

Ingredients:

Olive oil cooking spray
1   **(4-ounce) boneless skinless chicken cutlet**
    Kosher salt and fresh ground black pepper
½   **cup quartered water-packed artichoke hearts, drained**
1   **clove garlic, thinly sliced**
1   **cup washed spinach**
1½ **teaspoons chopped fresh rosemary**
½   **cup unsalted chicken stock (such as Kitchen Basics)**
    Lemon wedge, for serving

Method:

1. Spray a large nonstick skillet with cooking spray and place it over medium-high heat. Season the chicken lightly with salt and pepper and cook until browned on both sides, about 1 minute per side. Transfer to a plate and set aside.

2. Trim the leafy ends from the artichoke hearts and mince them. Set aside. Place the quartered artichoke hearts in the pan and cook until browned on the cut sides, about 5 minutes. Transfer the artichokes to the plate with the chicken. Add the minced artichoke leaves to the pan and cook until deeply browned, about 3 minutes (you may need to spray the pan again with cooking spray). Once browned, move the minced artichokes to the side of the pan, add the garlic, and cook, stirring, until golden brown, about 30 seconds. Add the spinach and cook until it has wilted, then transfer the mixture to a cutting board and finely chop it.

3. Return everything to the pan, add the chicken stock and rosemary, place over medium-high heat and simmer until the chicken is cooked through and the stock has reduced to coat everything, about 2 minutes. Season with salt and pepper and place the chicken on a plate, spoon the sauce and artichoke mixture evenly over the chicken dish, and serve with a lemon wedge.

Tip:

Add 2 cups of rinsed and dried shirataki rice or noodles to make this a super-filling dish for zero added calories.

Per serving:

176 calories, 1.5g fat (0.375g sat), 65.75mg cholesterol, 530mg sodium, 8.8g carbohydrate, 4.775g fiber, 30g protein

Recommended Ready-Made Version:

Lean Cuisine Baked Chicken
Fat: 7g / Calories: 240 cal

BEFORE

549 | 39.9
Calories | Fat

AFTER

176 | 1.5
Calories | Fat

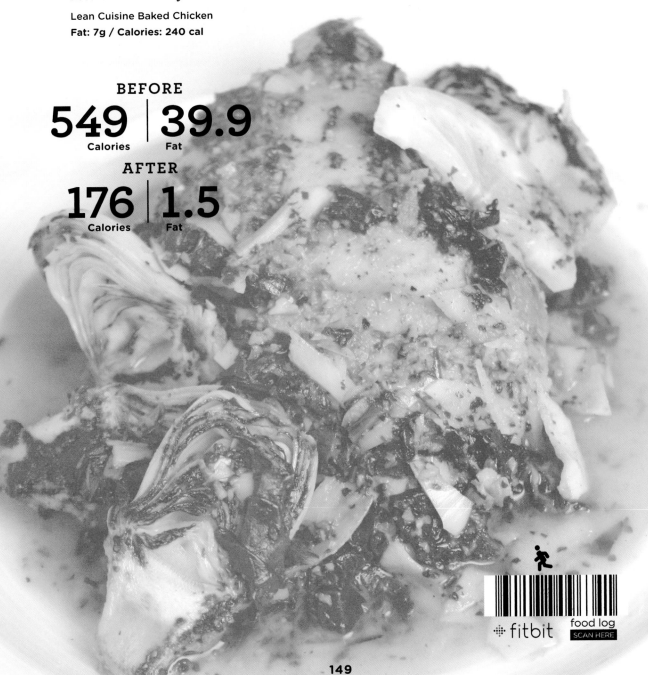

fitbit food log SCAN HERE

CHICKEN WITH MARINATED BEAN SPROUTS

HERE'S ANOTHER Asian-inspired dish you can whip up almost faster than the time it takes to read the recipe. Seriously, it doesn't take long to get it to the table—no longer than 25 minutes to fix. You've waited longer than that in a drive-through lane at dinnertime. Besides chicken cutlets, the main ingredient is bean sprouts. Rich in enzymes, sprouts help digestion and promote detoxification. Sprouts are alkaline in nature, too, for a more efficient metabolism and better immunity.

Yield	Prep time	Processing time	Calorie Burn	Calories	Net-Calories
1 main course	approximately 10 minutes	approximately 10 minutes	132	150	18

Ingredients:

	Olive oil cooking spray
½	poblano pepper
3	ounces boneless skinless chicken cutlets
	Kosher salt and freshly ground black pepper
1	cup bean sprouts
2	tablespoons sliced red onion
3	cherry tomatoes
⅛	teaspoon grated lime zest
1¼	teaspoons fresh lime juice
½	teaspoon fish sauce
½	teaspoon monk fruit crystals (such as Lakanto Golden Sweetener)
1	teaspoon green hot sauce (such as Tabasco Green Jalapeño)
4	fresh basil leaves
	Lime wedge, for serving

Method:

1. Spray a grill or grill pan with cooking spray and place it over high heat. Place the pepper on the grill and cook until charred on both sides. Meanwhile, season the chicken with salt and pepper and grill on both sides until fully cooked and lightly charred, about 2 minutes per side. Transfer the charred pepper and the chicken to a wire rack and let cool for 5 minutes. Transfer to a cutting board and cut both into strips.
2. Place the bean sprouts on a microwave-safe plate and microwave on high until they have just wilted, about 2 minutes. Run under cold water to cool and pat dry with a towel, then place in a bowl with the onion, tomatoes, lime zest, lime juice, fish sauce, monk fruit, and hot sauce. Add the pepper and chicken strips and the basil, toss, and season with salt and pepper.
3. Spoon the mixture onto a plate and garnish with lime.

Tip:

Add ½ cup fresh cilantro sprigs to this recipe for less than a calorie more.

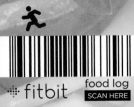

Per serving:

150 calories, 1.25 fat (0.325g sat), 49.25mg cholesterol, 301mg
sodium, 14.5g carbohydrate, 2.8g fiber, 23.7g protein

Recommended Ready-Made Version:

Lean Cuisine Sesame Chicken
Fat: 9g / Calories: 330 cal

BEFORE

325 | 12.3
Calories | Fat

AFTER

150 | 1.25
Calories | Fat

fitbit food log SCAN HERE

COOK YOUR BUTT OFF!

CHICKEN WITH PARSLEY, PEPPERS, AND LEMON

CHICKEN BREASTS aren't the sexiest protein around but they sure are popular for us waistline-watchers. Their popularity is matched only by their versatility. Because they have little flavor on their own, you can do almost anything with them. Pair chicken with herbs, spices, fruits, vegetables, or any number of other foods, and you have yourself a real meal. One of my favorite ways to enjoy chicken is to turn it into an exciting herb and vegetable dish like the one below.

Yield	Prep time	Processing time	Calorie Burn	Calories	Net-Calories
1 main course	approximately 15 minutes	approximately 15 minutes	121	194	73

Ingredients:

1	(4-ounce) boneless skinless chicken cutlet, halved lengthwise
	Kosher salt and freshly ground black pepper
	Olive oil cooking spray
½	cup medium-spicy peppers (such as poblanos), cut into bite-sized pieces
1	small Belgian endive, root end cut off and leaves separated
	Lemon wedge
¼	bunch fresh parsley, largest stems picked out and cut into 2-inch pieces
¼	teaspoon lemon zest

Method:

1. Preheat the oven to 350°F.
2. Place a cast-iron pan over high heat. Season the chicken with salt and black pepper and spray with cooking spray. Cook the chicken until blackened slightly on both sides, about 2 minutes per side, then transfer to a plate.
3. Place the hot peppers in the pan and cook until they are charred on all sides, about 2 minutes. Move the peppers to the side of the pan. Add half the endive to the pan, reduce the heat to low, and cook the endive until caramelized and softened, about 5 minutes. Place the lemon wedge cut-side down in the pan and place the chicken over the endive. Transfer the pan to the oven and bake until the chicken is cooked through, 3 to 5 minutes. Transfer the lemon wedge and chicken to a plate. Season the charred pepper and endive with salt and black pepper.
4. Chop the remaining endive into small pieces and mix with the charred peppers, cooked endive, parsley, and lemon zest. Season with salt and black pepper and plate next to the chicken breast. Squeeze the roasted pulp and juice from the cooked lemon over the top of the dish and serve.

Tips:

- Try adding 1 teaspoon fruity olive oil to the dressing on a special occasion for a luxurious perfume and an added 40 calories per salad.
- Add ¼ cup of your favorite herbs to this salad to give it a personal touch—try basil, cilantro, and chives!

Per serving:

194 calories, 2g fat (0.525g sat), 82.25mg cholesterol, 117.25mg sodium, 6.1g carbohydrate, 3.575g fiber, 34.65g protein

Recommended Ready-Made Version:

Lean Cuisine Herb Roasted Chicken
Fat: 4g / Calories: 180 cal

BEFORE

348 | **21**

Calories | Fat

AFTER

194 | **2**

Calories | Fat

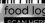

fitbit food log
SCAN HERE

153

COOK YOUR BUTT OFF!

CHILI-RUBBED CHICKEN WITH BLACK BEAN SALSA AND RICE

A "RUB" is a mixture of spices or herbs that is applied to food to give it flavor. A dry rub generally consists of spices, whereas a wet rub would consist of ingredients that are moist, such as juices and broths that form a paste that is applied to the food. Here, I use a simple dry rub of chili powder and salt for South of the Border pizzazz.

Yield	Prep time	Processing time	Calorie Burn	Calories	Net-Calories
1 main course	approximately 15 minutes	approximately 10 minutes	106	173	67

Ingredients:

Olive oil cooking spray

1 **(4-ounce) chicken breast cutlet**

Kosher salt and chili powder

½ **(7-ounce) bag shirataki rice (such as Miracle Rice), rinsed and drained**

½ **cup fresh pico de gallo (such as Ready Pac)**

2 **tablespoons drained no-salt-added black beans (such as Eden)**

¼ **cup fresh cilantro**

Method:

1. Spray a nonstick skillet with cooking spray and place it over medium-high heat. Season the chicken on both sides with salt and chili powder and cook on each side until browned and chicken is cooked through, about 2 minutes per side. Transfer to a plate and set aside.
2. Add the rice to the pan and cook until all of the water has evaporated, about 30 seconds. Transfer to a bowl with the pico de gallo and beans, mix well, and season with salt and chili powder.
3. Spoon the rice mixture into a bowl and top with the chicken and cilantro.

Tips:

- Serve this dish with fresh lime wedges for an added fresh burst for little to no added calories.
- Replace the Miracle Rice with ½ cup of defrosted frozen brown rice and add only 115 calories and 1g of fat.

Per serving:

173 calories, 1.5g fat (0.4g sat), 65.5mg cholesterol, 139mg sodium, 12.65g carbohydrate, 1.6g fiber, 27.9g protein

Recommended Ready-Made Version:

Lean Cuisine Santa Fe Rice and Beans
Fat: 5g / Calories: 290 cal

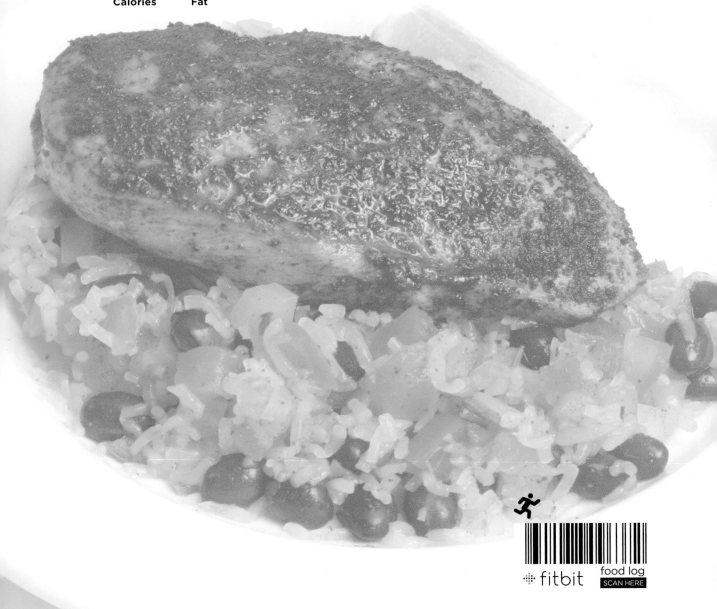

BEFORE

525 | **15**
Calories | Fat

AFTER

173 | **1.5**
Calories | Fat

fitbit food log
SCAN HERE

COD WITH TOMATOES, ZUCCHINI, AND BLACK OLIVES

I LOVE COD. It has a delicate flakiness, great texture, and natural sweetness. Many Greek and Italian restaurants feature it—which is where I got the inspiration for this delicious Mediterranean rendition with tomatoes, zucchini, basil, and black olives. In cod I trust!

Yield	Prep time	Processing time	Calorie Burn	Calories	Net-Calories
1 main course	**approximately 10 minutes**	**approximately 10 minutes**	**113**	**143**	**30**

Ingredients:

1	**small ripe tomato**
	Kosher salt
	Olive oil cooking spray
1	**(4-ounce) fillet fresh cod, haddock, or hake**
¼	**cup fresh basil leaves, roughly torn**
	Red pepper flakes
1	**cup grated zucchini**
2	**pitted oil-cured black olives, roughly chopped**

Method:

1. Cut the tomato in half. Press the cut side of each half against the large holes of a box grater and grate while pushing on the skin with your palm. This should yield ¼ cup of pulp. Place the pulp in a small bowl, season with salt, and set aside.
2. Spray a large nonstick skillet with cooking spray and place it over medium-high heat. Season the fish with salt on both flat sides and cook until browned. Flip the fillet and cook for about 1 minute more.
3. Season the fish and add the basil and red pepper flakes to the pan to wilt, then add the zucchini and olives, reduce the heat to medium, cover, and simmer until the fish is cooked through, about 1 minute.
4. Spoon the zucchini on a plate. Place the fillet on top, add black olives, and pour the tomato pulp around the fish. Serve.

Tip:

Try adding ¼ teaspoon grated orange zest to this recipe for an interesting perfume and next to no calories.

Per serving:

143 calories, 2g fat (1.175g sat), 48.75mg cholesterol, 184mg sodium, 8.7g carbohydrate, 2.2g fiber, 22.25g protein

Recommended Ready-Made Version:

Lean Cuisine Lemon Pepper Fish
Fat: 8g / Calories: 300 cal

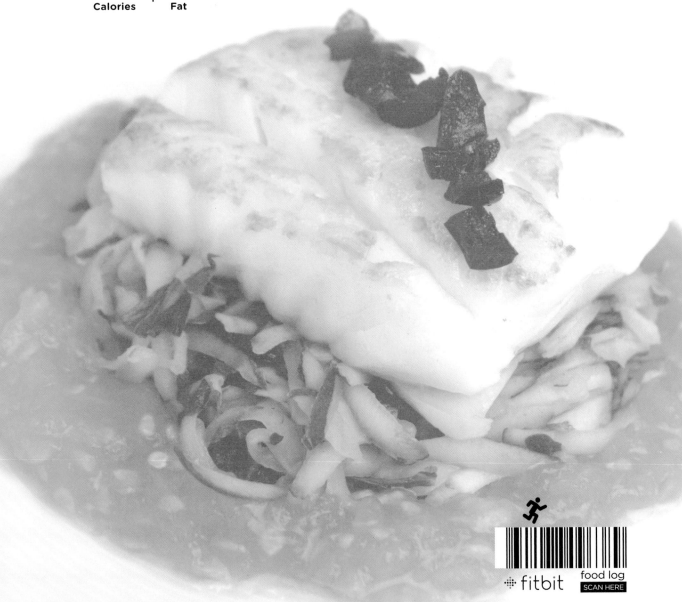

BEFORE

328 | 14
Calories | **Fat**

AFTER

143 | 2
Calories | **Fat**

fitbit food log
SCAN HERE

COOK YOUR BUTT OFF!

MEAT LOAF WITH MASHED SWEET POTATOES

MEAT LOAF is true comfort food no matter how you slice it—and downsizing comfort food is my favorite cooking challenge. In this recipe, I've used puffed brown rice in place of high-carb, low-nutrition bread crumbs to reduce the calories. What's more, I reduced the amount of meat traditionally used in a meat loaf recipe. If you're new to cooking, meat loaf is something you cannot screw up. It's just about the most forgiving recipe you'll ever make. Adding a little more of this or a little less of that usually doesn't make a heck of a difference in the end. What you have, too, is a full-flavored and meaty meat loaf that tastes substantial, a savory classic dish so good that it might even taste like the one your mom or grandma used to make.

Yield	Prep time	Processing time	Calorie Burn	Calories	Net-Calories
1 main course	approximately 15 minutes	approximately 15 minutes	141	175.5	34.5

Ingredients:

1   small sweet potato, peeled and grated on large holes of a box grater (about ¾ cups)
2   tablespoons water
    Kosher salt and freshly ground black pepper
½   cup puffed brown rice
¼   cup fat-free reduced-sodium chicken stock (such as Kitchen Basics)
3   ounces 96% lean ground beef (such as Laura's Lean)
1½ teaspoons egg white powder (such as Deb El Just Whites)
1   tablespoon no-sugar-added ketchup (such as AlternaSweets)

Method:

1. Preheat the oven to 400°F.
2. Place the grated sweet potatoes on a large microwave-safe plate and stir in the water. Season with salt and pepper, cover with waxed or parchment paper, and microwave on high until soft and fully cooked, about 5 minutes. Set aside.
3. Meanwhile, combine the puffed brown rice, stock, beef, and egg white powder in a large bowl and using a heavy-duty whisk, beat the mixture together until you have one homogenous mass. Season with salt and pepper. Spoon the mixture into a small six-inch nonstick ovenproof skillet into a flat layer about 1 inch thick. Place the pan over medium-high heat and begin to cook while evenly spreading the ketchup over the top. Transfer the pan to the oven on the middle rack and bake until the meat loaf is cooked through, about 5 minutes.
4. Remove the meat loaf from the skillet, slice it, and place it on a plate. Spoon the sweet potatoes next to the slices and serve.

Tips:

- If you like a real caramelized glaze on the meat loaf, turn the oven to broil for the last 2 minutes of cooking.
- You can cook this meat loaf in ceramic bakeware as well and skip the stovetop cooking. Add 5 to 10 minutes cooking time in the oven depending on the shape of the bakeware chosen.

Per serving:

175.5 calories, 3.5g fat (0.75g sat, 0g mono, 0g poly), 45mg cholesterol, 269.25mg sodium, 10.7g carbohydrate, 1.15g fiber, 20.25g protein

Recommended Ready-Made Version:

Healthy Choice Classic Meat Loaf
Fat: 8g / Calories: 350 cal

BEFORE

670 | **42**
Calories | Fat

AFTER

175.5 | **3.5**
Calories | Fat

fitbit food log
SCAN HERE

PUMPKIN RISOTTO WITH SAGE

MY FAVORITE cheese for lean, healthy cooking is Parmigiano-Reggiano, which you'll find in this delightful risotto, a classic Italian dish made with rice and other ingredients. This cheese has an impressive résumé, from being high in protein and low in fat to being quickly absorbed by the body for energy. I recently learned it's a great choice if you're lactose intolerant. Six to eight hours after Parmigiano-Reggiano is produced, its lactose is altered by natural enzymes in the cheese into an easily digestible lactic acid. Many lactose intolerant people can thus tolerate Parmigiano-Reggiano in moderate amounts. Everyone's tolerance is different, so please consult your physician before consuming Parmigiano-Reggiano if you are lactose intolerant. One more thing: I use shirataki rice here. It is gluten-free and carb free, but definitely not free of flavor!

Yield	Prep time	Processing time	Calorie Burn	Calories	Net-Calories
1 main course	approximately 10 minutes	approximately 15 minutes	170	138.5	-31.5

Ingredients:

1	cup grated butternut squash or pumpkin
	Olive oil cooking spray
1	(7-ounce) bag shirataki rice (such as Miracle Rice), rinsed and dried
1	tablespoon chopped fresh sage leaves
1¼	cups store-cut mixed wild mushrooms
½	cup unsalted fat-free chicken stock
1	scant teaspoon arrowroot powder
¼	ounce Parmigiano-Reggiano, grated with a Microplane
	Kosher salt and freshly ground black pepper

Method:

1. Place the grated squash into a microwave-safe bowl, cover with a microwave-safe plate, and microwave on high until tender, about 4 minutes. Set aside.
2. Spray a large nonstick skillet with cooking spray and place it over medium-high heat. Add the rice and cook until all the water has evaporated, about 30 seconds. Remove the rice and set aside. Spray the pan again with cooking spray, add half the sage and mushrooms, and cook until the mushrooms have softened, about 2 minutes.
3. Add the rice, cooked squash, and three-quarters of the stock to the pan and bring to a simmer. Combine the remaining stock and arrowroot powder in a small bowl and add it to the risotto, stirring until the risotto becomes thick, about 30 seconds. Reduce the heat to low and add three-quarters of the Parmigiano and the remaining sage and stir until the risotto is smooth. Season with salt and pepper.
4. Spoon the risotto into a bowl, evenly distribute the remaining Parmigiano over the dish, and serve.

Tips:

- If you want to boost the sweetness of the dish, try adding just ½ teaspoon monk fruit crystals (such as Lakanto Golden Sweetener) for no additional calories.
- Substitute the Miracle Rice with ¾ cup of cooked short grain brown rice (check the freezer section or buy from Asian take out) and add 164 calories and just over 1 gram of fat.

Per serving:

138.5 calories, 2.5g fat (1.55g sat), 6.25mg cholesterol, 110mg sodium, 24.6g carbohydrate, 4.38g fiber, 9.2g protein

Recommended Ready-Made Version:

Domo Risotto with Chicken and Merken
Fat: 0.5g / Calories: 160 cal

BEFORE

405 | 10.5
Calories | Fat

AFTER

138.5 | 2.5
Calories | Fat

fitbit food log
SCAN HERE

ASIAN PORK BUNS

USUALLY THIS dish is made with fattening pork belly and high-gluten bread flour. But here, I've kept the fat on the pig (by using lean pork loin) and the gluten in the pantry. That way, you can enjoy this dish and feel great afterward, especially with a side of fresh ginger slaw! Plus, it takes no time to prepare, since the pork is precooked from the deli.

Yield	Prep time	Processing time	Calorie Burn	Calories	Net-Calories
2 buns	approximately 15 minutes	approximately 15 minutes	157	182	25

Ingredients:

1 tablespoon all-natural prune baby food (such as Gerber 1st Foods All Natural)

1 teaspoon gluten-free reduced-sodium tamari (such as San-J)

2 teaspoons monk fruit crystals (such as Lakanto Golden Sweetener)

½ teaspoon white wine vinegar, plus ¼ cup for rinsing

¼ teaspoon finely grated peeled fresh ginger (grated on a Microplane)

¼ cup thinly sliced, unpeeled cucumbers

Kosher salt

52 grams frozen gluten-free pizza dough, cut into 2 equal pieces

1 ounce store-roasted pork loin, trimmed of all visible fat and thinly sliced at your deli

¼ cup fresh cilantro sprigs

Method:

1. Place a steamer on the stove and bring to a simmer. In a small bowl, mix together the prunes, tamari, monk fruit, ½ teaspoon vinegar, and the ginger and set aside.

2. Lay the cucumber slices out in a single layer on a baking sheet, lightly sprinkle each side with salt, and let stand for 5 minutes. Rinse off the salt with the remaining ¼ cup vinegar, shake off the excess, and set aside.

3. Place each piece of pizza dough between two pieces of plastic wrap and roll into round discs ¼ inch thick. Place each disc on a piece of waxed paper and place them in the steamer (not touching each other). Steam until they are cooked through, about 2 minutes. Remove, fold one side over the other crosswise, and set aside under a warm towel.

4. Spoon half the prune mixture into a saucepan with the pork, place the pan over medium heat, and fold the pork together with the sauce until hot. Remove from the heat.

5. Spoon the remaining prune sauce inside each bun, evenly distribute the pork and cucumbers between the buns, then fold over one side of the buns to enclose the filling. Place the buns on a plate, top with cilantro, and serve.

Tips:

• Add 1 leaf of butter lettuce to each bun for an extra calorie per serving.

• Add some thinly sliced raw jalapeños and scallions to spice things up a bit for about a calorie extra per serving.

Per serving:

182 calories, 4g fat (0.33g sat, 0g mono, 0g poly), 20.6mg cholesterol, 393mg sodium, 26.75g carbohydrate, 0.55g fiber, 11.2g protein

Recommended Ready-Made Version:

Chef Hon Steamed Pork Buns
Fat: 4g / Calories: 180 cal

BEFORE

440 | **31**
Calories | Fat

AFTER

182 | **4**
Calories | Fat

fitbit food log SCAN HERE

ROASTED PORK WITH SAUERKRAUT, APPLES, AND DIJON MUSTARD

THE PAIRING of roasted pork and apples is nothing new, but delivering it in twenty minutes and around 220 calories per serving is! Time-wise, dinner is one place where you can take the easy way out. You can't half wash the clothes, or partially clean the dishes, but you can take plenty of shortcuts in cooking, and that's what I've done here. Although you can use any type of apple, I've chosen the Gala variety for this recipe. They're juicy, crisp, hugely flavorful, and readily available all year long . Plus, they cook up tender and sweet. Pink Lady apples are a good alternative.

Yield	Prep time	Processing time	Calorie Burn	Calories	Net-Calories
1 main course	approximately 5 minutes	approximately 20 minutes	110	220	110

Ingredients:

Olive oil cooking spray

4 ounces trimmed pork tenderloin, cut into 2 medallions

Kosher salt and freshly ground black pepper

1 small Gala apple, cored

1½ teaspoons smooth (not whole-grain) Dijon mustard

6 tablespoons sliced onions

½ cup "live" sauerkraut, like Rejuvenate

Method:

1. Preheat the oven to 350°F.
2. Spray a nonstick ovenproof skillet with cooking spray and place it over medium-high heat. Season the medallions with salt and pepper on both sides and once the pan is hot, place them in the pan. Cook until browned on each side, about 2 minutes per side, then transfer to a plate and set aside.
3. Slice half of the apple into ¼-inch slices and set aside. Using a Microplane or the small holes of a box grater, grate the other half into a bowl and mix in the mustard. Put the onions and sliced apples in the pan, reduce the heat to medium, and cook, stirring, until the apples and onions have softened, 7 to 10 minutes. Place the pork on top of the onions and apples and place in the oven to finish cooking the pork, 2 to 5 minutes.
4. Transfer the pork to a plate. Add the sauerkraut to the pan with the onions and apples and toss to warm. Evenly distribute the mixture next to and under the pork.
5. Dollop the apple mustard on top of the pork and serve.

Tip:

- Add 1 teaspoon chopped fresh thyme to this recipe for added aroma and next to no calories.
- "Live" sauerkraut means it was not heated and all the microflora were not destroyed so they are available to your body.

Per serving:

220 calories, 4.5g fat (1.35g sat, 0g mono, 0g poly), 73.75mg cholesterol, 353mg sodium, 18g carbohydrate, 7.8g fiber, 25.5g protein

Recommended Ready-Made Version:

Lean Cuisine Herb Roasted Chicken
Fat: 4g / Calories: 180 cal

BEFORE

590 | **33**
Calories | Fat

AFTER

220 | **4.5**
Calories | Fat

fitbit food log
SCAN HERE

GRILLED HEARTS OF ROMAINE WITH MARINATED SHRIMP

IF YOU haven't already met, let me introduce you to a terrific summery dinner. You'll actually be grilling lettuce, along with shrimp. This might sound odd, but the flavor of grilled lettuce certainly is not. Multiply the recipe for a crowd.

Yield	Prep time	Processing time	Calorie Burn	Calories	Net-Calories
1 serving	approximately 10 minutes	approximately 12 minutes	142	95	-47

Ingredients:

1	romaine lettuce heart, halved lengthwise
2	ounces peeled and cleaned medium shrimp (6 shrimp)
	Kosher salt and freshly ground black pepper
	Olive oil cooking spray
¼	cup chopped fresh tomatoes
¼	cup chopped jícama
¼	teaspoon grated lime zest
2	teaspoons fresh lime juice
¼	cup fresh cilantro, chopped
	Lime wedges, for serving

Method:

1. Preheat a grill or grill pan to medium-high heat. Cut the romaine lettuce into six two-inch chunks and skewer with the shrimp alternating between lettuce and shrimp. Chop the remaining lettuce. Season the skewers with salt and pepper on both sides, spray with cooking spray and place on the grill and cook until the shrimp is cooked and the lettuce is lightly charred, about 1 to 2 minutes per side. Flip and grill on the other side, about 1 minute more.
2. Combine the remaining ingredients in a bowl and season with salt and pepper.
3. Place the grilled skewers on a plate and evenly spoon the tomato mixture over the top. Serve with lime wedges.

Tips:

- Mix 1 tablespoon lime juice with 1 tablespoon plain fat-free Greek yogurt for a creamy addition to each salad for 13 calories and zero fat.
- If you find yourself pressed for time, skip the grilling and just chop the romaine hearts for a fast and delicious salad.

Per serving:

95 calories, 0.5g fat (0.175g sat), 110mg cholesterol, 110mg sodium, 8.6g carbohydrate, 13.6g fiber, 4.3g protein

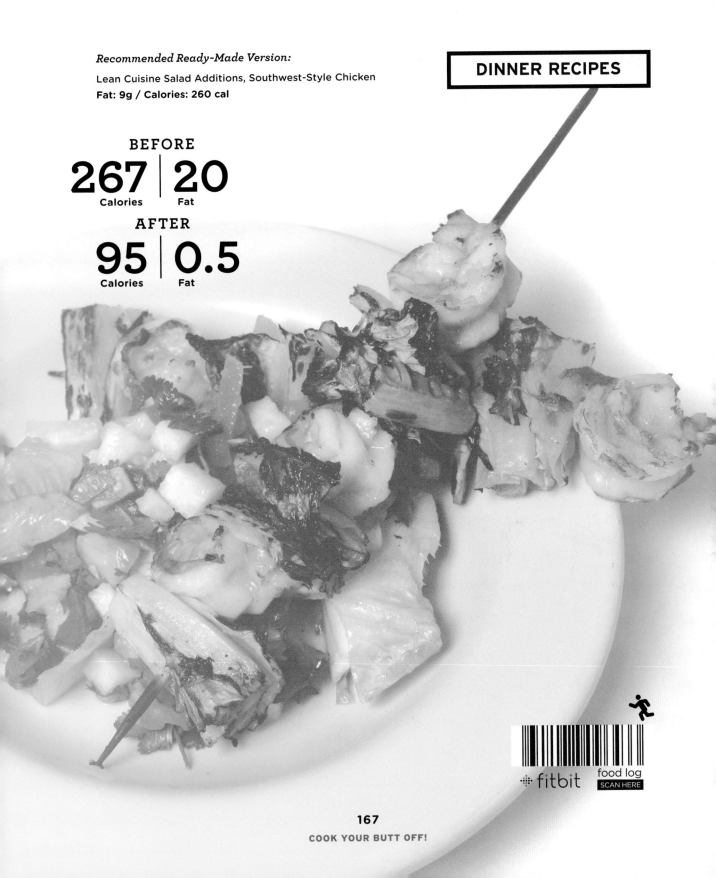

Recommended Ready-Made Version:

Lean Cuisine Salad Additions, Southwest-Style Chicken
Fat: 9g / Calories: 260 cal

BEFORE
267 | 20
Calories | Fat

AFTER
95 | 0.5
Calories | Fat

DINNER RECIPES

fitbit food log SCAN HERE

COOK YOUR BUTT OFF!

SOY SPAGHETTI WITH SHRIMP AND HAND-CHOPPED POMODORO SAUCE

TO WHIP up something delicious, quick, and healthy, try this recipe. I've used a very healthy pasta alternative, made from soy, low-calorie boiled shrimp, and red pepper flakes for a metabolism boost. This full-flavored dish will have everyone around the table singing "That's Amore."

Yield	Prep time	Processing time	Calorie Burn	Calories	Net-Calories
1 main course	approximately 10 minutes	approximately 15 minutes	115	185	70

Ingredients:

Kosher salt

1 **ounce gluten-free soy spaghetti (such as Explore Asia)**

Olive oil cooking spray

2 **teaspoons finely chopped garlic**

2 **ounces peeled domestic white shrimp, halved lengthwise**

Red pepper flakes

¼ **cup packed fresh basil leaves, torn into small pieces**

¾ **cup chopped fresh tomatoes**

½ **teaspoon finely chopped capers**

Method:

1. In a wide saucepan with a lid, bring 2 quarts of water to a boil over high heat. Add 2 teaspoons of salt, drop in the spaghetti, and set a timer for 5 minutes. Drain and set aside.
2. Meanwhile, spray a large nonstick skillet for 4 seconds with cooking spray and place it over medium-high heat. Add the garlic and cook until golden brown, then add the shrimp, red pepper flakes to taste, and the basil and cook until the basil has wilted, about 30 seconds.
3. Remove the shrimp, add the tomatoes and capers to the pan, and bring to a simmer. Break up the tomatoes with a wooden spoon and cook until the sauce has the texture of marinara sauce. Return the shrimp to the pan and add the cooked pasta. Simmer and toss until the pasta is tender and the shrimp are warmed through, about 1 minute. Plate the pasta and shrimp in a pasta bowl and serve.

Tips:

- If you don't eat shrimp, you can substitute cooked boneless skinless chicken breast for an additional 17 calories per serving.
- Make it a super-filling and healthy "primavera" dish by adding a frozen steamed vegetable blend for only 40 calories per ¾ cup.
- You can substitute shirataki penne and save 127 calories per portion!

Per serving:

185 calories, 2g fat (.7g sat, 0g mono, 0g poly), 86.25mg cholesterol, 147.5mg sodium, 16.425g carbohydrate, 7.4g fiber, 24.7g protein

Recommended Ready-Made Version:

Smart Ones Shrimp Marinara
Fat: 2.5g / Calories: 180 cal

BEFORE
1240 | **72**
Calories | Fat

AFTER
185 | **2**
Calories | Fat

fitbit food log
SCAN HERE

COOK YOUR BUTT OFF!

SPAGHETTI WITH ASPARAGUS PESTO AND PECORINO ROMANO

I LOVE pesto and could eat a whole jarful with my finger. Unfortunately, this puree of basil, olive oil, garlic, and pine nuts packs serious fat and calories. In this recipe, pureed asparagus is a light alternative to conventional versions and a great veggie base for pesto because it has a powerful flavor. Combined with a bit of raw garlic, it creates a pesto that is fresh and memorable. I puree it with a tiny amount of olive oil and only a few tablespoons of grated low-lactose Pecorino Romano. The resulting pesto is lighter than most and makes delicious sauce for pasta.

Yield	Prep time	Processing time	Calorie Burn	Calories	Net-Calories
1 main course	**approximately 15 minutes**	**approximately 10 minutes**	**161**	**208.5**	**47.5**

Ingredients:

12	ounces fresh asparagus
½	teaspoon plus ¼ teaspoon extra virgin olive oil
¼	teaspoon minced garlic
½	cup fresh basil leaves
	Kosher salt
1¼	ounces gluten-free corn spaghetti (such as Mrs. Leeper's)
¼	ounce freshly grated Pecorino Romano
	Freshly ground black pepper

Method:

1. Place the asparagus on a cutting board and trim the tough ends so you have 4-inch spears. Slice the spears lengthwise as thin as possible and reserve. Place the olive oil in a nonstick skillet over medium-high heat. Once the pan is hot, add the chopped asparagus ends and garlic and fry until the asparagus turns green and fragrant. Add the basil and cook until just wilted. Transfer the asparagus mixture to a cutting board and chop until it forms a fine paste.

2. Bring 4 quarts of water to a boil in a saucepan. Add 1 tablespoon salt and add the pasta. Stir the pasta until all the noodles are separated. Cook for 4 minutes. Add the sliced asparagus and cook until the pasta is al dente and the asparagus is tender, about 3 minutes. Drain the noodles, rinse under warm water and reserve 2 tablespoons of cooking liquid, and set both aside.

3. Return the pasta, asparagus spears, asparagus paste, and 1 tablespoon of the cooking liquid to the pan, set over medium heat to warm through, and toss to coat. Turn off the heat and add three-quarters of the cheese. Season with salt and pepper and toss to coat so everything is just sticking to the spaghetti. Plate the pasta in a bowl and top with the remaining cheese.

Tips:

- Add 1 tablespoon toasted chopped walnuts to this dish for a little texture and authentic feel for an additional 47 calories per serving.
- Feel free to use Parmigiano Reggiano instead of Pecorino Romano for a more classic pesto flavor.

Per serving:

208.5 calories, 5.5g fat (2.25g sat), 4.75mg cholesterol, 110mg sodium, 35g carbohydrate, 4.7g fiber, 6.8g protein

BEFORE

798 | 38
Calories | Fat

AFTER

208.5 | 5.5
Calories | Fat

fitbit food log SCAN HERE

COOK YOUR BUTT OFF!

SPINACH DUMPLINGS WITH MARINARA

HERE'S A DISH that would make Popeye proud. Spinach is a true superfood, loaded with vitamins, minerals, antioxidants, and phytochemicals that keep you healthy. For this reason, I love to use spinach in as many recipes as I can.

Yield	Prep time	Processing time	Calorie Burn	Calories	Net-Calories
1 main course	approximately 20 minutes	approximately 10 minutes	117	126	9

Ingredients:

Olive oil cooking spray

2 small cloves garlic, chopped

¼ bunch fresh basil (about 10 leaves)

Red pepper flakes

5 ounces washed spinach

1 tablespoon egg white powder

Kosher salt

½ cup no-sugar-added fat-free marinara (such as Colavita)

3 grams grated Parmigiano-Reggiano (optional)

Method:

1. Spray a nonstick skillet with cooking spray, place it over medium-high heat, and add the garlic. Cook the garlic, stirring, until it is golden brown. Add the basil, a pinch of red pepper flakes, and the spinach. Cook until the spinach has wilted and the water has evaporated out of it when you press on it with a spatula. The spinach must be fully cooked with all excess water evaporated.

2. Place the spinach mixture on a cutting board and chop very fine. Place in a bowl (set over a bowl of ice water, if still hot) and whisk in the egg white powder until it has dissolved; there can be no lumps. Season with salt.

3. Pour the marinara into a microwave-safe serving vessel and using a tablespoon measure, make 5 dollops of the spinach mixture in the sauce. Cover with parchment paper and microwave on high until the dumplings are set, about 2 minutes. Serve topped with the Parmigiano, if desired.

Tips:

Sprinkle each dish with ¼ ounce Parmigiano-Reggiano for an additional 28 calories. Most lactose-intolerant people can have Parmigiano-Reggiano, but please consult your physician first.

Per serving:

126 calories, 4.5g fat (0.75g sat, 0g mono, 0g poly), 2.75mg cholesterol, 527mg sodium, 18.65g carbohydrate, 6.2g fiber, 11.8g protein

BEFORE

252 | **9**
Calories | Fat

AFTER

126 | **4.5**
Calories | Fat

fitbit food log SCAN HERE

COOK YOUR BUTT OFF!

SWEET POTATO SPAETZLE

SPAETZLE–WHAT'S that you ask? It's basically a European dumpling with roots in Germany and Austria. My dumplings get their body from the luscious sweet potato, which yields a light, supple spaetzle that can stand with the best. A serving supplies 13 grams of fat-fighting fiber and 18 grams of protein, making it a superfood.

Yield	Prep time	Processing time	Calorie Burn	Calories	Net-Calories
1 main course	approximately 15 minutes	approximately 15 minutes	121	205	84

Ingredients:

Kosher salt

1 cup grated sweet potatoes

1 tablespoon cold water

2 tablespoons psyllium husk powder

3½ tablespoons egg white powder

Freshly grated nutmeg

Olive oil cooking spray

3 large fresh sage leaves, roughly chopped

¾ cup washed spinach

½ cup chicken stock

Grated Parmigiano-Reggiano, for serving (optional)

Method:

1. Bring 6 quarts of water to a boil in a large saucepan and add 2 tablespoons salt.
2. Place the sweet potatoes, cold water, and psyllium in a blender and blend until smooth and thickened, about 1 minute. Add the egg white powder and season with salt and nutmeg. Blend until the egg white powder has dissolved, about 30 seconds.
3. Using a potato ricer, colander, or any utensil with small holes, begin to push the sweet potato mixture through the holes with a rubber spatula directly into the boiling water. Let the spaetzle cook until they float to the top, about 10 seconds. Scoop them out with a slotted spoon and place in a colander to drain. Shake off any excess water. Repeat until all the spaetzle is cooked.
4. Spray a large nonstick skillet with cooking spray and place it over medium-high heat. Once the pan is hot, add the spaetzle and cook until lightly browned. Add the sage, cook for 5 seconds, and then add the spinach. Cook until the spinach has wilted, then add the chicken stock and cook until it has thickened slightly. Spoon the spaetzle into a bowl and serve with Parmigiano, if desired.

Per serving:

205 calories, 0g fat (0g sat), 70mg cholesterol, 399mg sodium, 37g carbohydrate, 13.5g fiber, 18.75g protein

BEFORE
321 | 6.4
Calories | Fat

AFTER
205 | 0
Calories | Fat

fitbit food log
SCAN HERE

COOK YOUR BUTT OFF!

VEGETABLE FRIED "RICE"

I'VE REPLACED rice with cauliflower here to lose the carbs. You might be turning up your nose at the cauliflower—it isn't the most popular veggie on the produce block, for reasons unknown. But I suspect cauliflower is low in popularity partly because we don't have many ideas for what to do with it, except for maybe drenching it in fattening cheese sauce. But here, I cook it in such a way that it tastes better than rice!

Yield	Prep time	Processing time	Calorie Burn	Calories	Net-Calories
1 main course	approximately 2 minutes	approximately 10 minutes	172	105	-67

Ingredients:

Olive oil cooking spray

Pinch of red pepper flakes, plus more as desired

½ head cauliflower, grated on the small holes of box grater to the size of rice (about 1 cup)

Kosher salt

2 cups fresh stir-fry vegetable medley (look in produce department for a mix with broccoli, peppers, mushrooms, onions, snap peas, bean sprouts, etc.), chopped into ½-inch pieces

¾ teaspoon chopped garlic

½ teaspoon chopped peeled fresh ginger

1 teaspoon gluten-free, reduced-sodium tamari (such as San-J)

Method:

1. Spray a large nonstick skillet with cooking spray and place it over medium-high heat. Add the red pepper flakes and grated cauliflower and cook until the cauliflower is lightly browned, about 30 seconds. Season with salt, transfer to a bowl, and set aside.

2. Spray the pan again with cooking spray and add the vegetables. Cook until the vegetables are charred and softened, about 1 minute. Move the vegetables to one side of the pan and add the garlic and ginger to the exposed part of the pan. Cook until aromatic, about 20 seconds. Return the cauliflower "rice" to the pan and toss until everything is well mixed. Turn off the heat, add the tamari, and toss the mixture until everything is well coated. Season with salt and more red pepper flakes, if desired.

3. Spoon the mixture into a bowl and serve.

Tips:

• Add 2 ounces cooked and shredded chicken for an added 95 protein-packed calories per dish.
• Add one egg after the garlic and ginger is cooked and scramble it to turn this into a great breakfast for an added 54 calories and 4g of fat.
• Serve with chopped fresh cilantro and lime juice for a burst of freshness.

Per serving:

105 calories, 0g fat (0.05g sat), 0mg cholesterol, 292mg sodium, 23.1g carbohydrate, 7.75g fiber, 7.55g protein

Recommended Ready-Made Version:

Lean Cuisine Chicken Fried Rice

Fat: 3g / Calories: 230 cal

BEFORE

405 | 20
Calories | **Fat**

AFTER

105 | 0
Calories | **Fat**

fitbit food log SCAN HERE

BLT Salad

Chopped Salad with Shrimp and Creamy Cilantro-Lime Dressing

Creamy Asian-style Slaw with Salmon

Salad with Carrot-Ginger Dressing

Heart of Palm and Escarole Salad with Spicy Oranges and Avocado

Cauliflower and Kale Salad with Lemon

Lentil Salad with Sherry Vinegar and Mirepoix

CHAPTER 10

Salad and Soup Recipes

Fresh Pea Salad with Smoked Salmon and Creamy Horseradish Dressing

Grilled Turkey Cutlet with Pear, Arugula, and Sprout Salad with Avocado

Kimchi-Cucumber Salad with Apples and Shaved Pork

Cream of Mushroom Soup

Hot-and-Sour Noodle Soup with Mushrooms

BLT SALAD

I'M A sucker for a good ol' BLT with thick-cut bacon, leafy green lettuce, juicy sliced tomatoes, and gobs of mayo—and plenty of calories and fat. That's why I definitely had to reinvent the classic BLT and turn it into a salad. You get all the taste of a BLT but none of the fattening stuff. This is a gluten-free dish, too.

Yield	Prep time	Processing time	Calorie Burn	Calories	Net-Calories
1 salad	approximately 8 minutes	approximately 15 minutes	58	140	82

Ingredients:

½	slice gluten-free multigrain bread (such as Udi's)
1	tablespoon light canola mayonnaise (such as Spectrum)
½	teaspoon fresh lemon juice
2	cups iceberg lettuce, torn into large bite-sized pieces
4	torn fresh basil leaves
1	cup cherry tomatoes, halved
	Kosher salt and freshly ground black pepper
2	tablespoons real bacon bits (such as Hormel)

Method:

1. Toast the bread in a toaster until golden brown and then tear it into bite-sized pieces. Keep warm.
2. In a medium bowl, whisk together the mayonnaise and lemon juice. Add the lettuce, basil, and tomatoes, and toss to coat evenly with dressing. Season with salt and pepper.
3. Sprinkle the bacon bits and toast pieces over the salad and serve.

Per serving:

140 calories, 6g fat (0.05g sat), 25mg cholesterol, 420mg sodium, 14g carbohydrate, 3.2g fiber, 9g protein

Recommended Ready-Made Version:

Chop't Salad with romaine lettuce, turkey, tomatoes, and Spa Dijon dressing
Fat: 6g / Calories: 255 cal

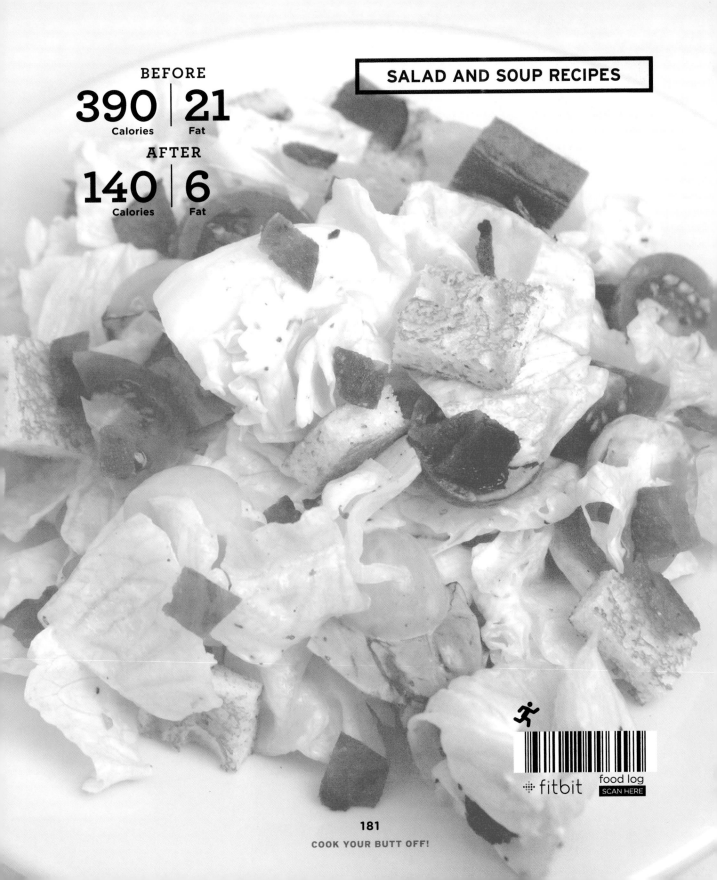

BEFORE

390 | **21**
Calories | Fat

AFTER

140 | **6**
Calories | Fat

SALAD AND SOUP RECIPES

fitbit food log
SCAN HERE

CHOPPED SALAD WITH SHRIMP AND CREAMY CILANTRO-LIME DRESSING

IF YOU think I'm into shrimp, you're right. This super-fresh-tasting salad is a real rock star! It is super low in calories and a great example of how simple preparations are best. You can even select your own favorite cruciferous vegetables and hand chop them yourself.

Yield	Prep time	Processing time	Calorie Burn	Calories	Net-Calories
1 salad	approximately 5 minutes	approximately 5 minutes	93	98	5

Ingredients:

½   **heaping cup fresh cilantro sprigs**
¼   **teaspoon grated lime zest**
1   **tablespoon fresh strained lime juice**
     Kosher salt
     Cayenne pepper
1   **tablespoon unsweetened cultured coconut milk (such as So Delicious)**
1½   **cups store-prepared fresh vegetable medley (cabbage, broccoli, cauliflower, bell peppers, etc.)**
½   **ounce cooked, peeled, and deveined shrimp**
     Lime wedge, for serving

Method:

1. Place three-quarters of the cilantro into a mortar with the lime zest and smash with the pestle into a fine paste. In a large bowl, whisk together the lime juice, a small pinch each of salt and cayenne, and the coconut milk until creamy, about 20 seconds. Add the cilantro paste to the bowl and whisk.
2. Place the vegetable medley on a cutting board and chop into ½-inch pieces. Chop the shrimp into 1-inch pieces and add the shrimp and vegetables to the bowl with the cilantro mixture.
3. Season and toss the salad to coat everything evenly, spoon into a salad bowl, top with the remaining cilantro sprigs, and serve with a lime wedge.

Tips:

- Try adding a few drops of jalapeño hot sauce or thinly sliced fresh jalapeños for great kick to your palate and metabolism.
- For an added coconut punch and ultra creamy texture, whisk ½ teaspoon of unrefined coconut oil into the dressing for an added 20 calories and 2½ grams of fat.

Per serving:

98 calories, 1g fat (0.2g sat), 83mg cholesterol, 137mg sodium, 9.26g carbohydrate, 3.175g fiber, 11.1g protein

Recommended Ready-Made Version:

Chop't Salad, with romaine, broccoli, bell peppers, and Spa Tex-Mex dressing
Fat: 1.5g / Calories: 155 cal

BEFORE

348 | **10**
Calories | Fat

AFTER

98 | **1**
Calories | Fat

fitbit food log
SCAN HERE

COOK YOUR BUTT OFF!

CREAMY ASIAN-STYLE SLAW WITH SALMON

HERE'S AN Asian twist on a classic: American barbecued ribs. Salmon subs for the ribs! And what a sub it is. Salmon is so versatile; it does everything in the kitchen except run the dishwasher. You can pair it with just about any sauce, and the dish always comes out a winner.

Yield	Prep time	Processing time	Calorie Burn	Calories	Net-Calories
1 salad	approximately 10 minutes	approximately 15 minutes	96	198	102

Ingredients:

1½   tablespoons plain fat-free Greek yogurt (such as Fage 0%)
⅛   teaspoon grated lime zest
2¼   teaspoons fresh lime juice
½   teaspoon minced red jalapeño
½   bunch broccoli, stems removed and peeled and cut into matchstick-sized pieces (1 cup)
¼   head red cabbage, cut into matchstick-sized pieces (½ cup)
2   tablespoons lightly chopped fresh cilantro
  Kosher salt
½   packet monk fruit extract (such as Monk Fruit in the Raw)
3   ounces skinless salmon fillet
  Olive oil cooking spray
  Lime wedge, for serving

Method:

1. In a medium bowl, combine the yogurt, lime zest, lime juice, jalapeño, broccoli, cabbage, and cilantro, and season with salt and monk fruit. Set aside.
2. Season the salmon with salt. Spray a cast iron pan with cooking spray and place over medium high heat. Once the pan is hot, add the salmon and cook until dark brown on each side and warmed through, about two minutes per side.
3. Spoon the slaw onto a plate, top with the salmon, and serve with a lime wedge.

Per serving:

198 calories, 7.5g fat,(0g sat fat), 20mg cholesterol, 113mg sodium, 9.5g carbohydrate, 3g fiber, 23.5g protein

Recommended Ready-Made Version:

Lean Cuisine Salmon with Basil
Fat: 6g / Calories: 210 cal

BEFORE

1,105 | 94
Calories Fat

AFTER

198 | 7.5
Calories Fat

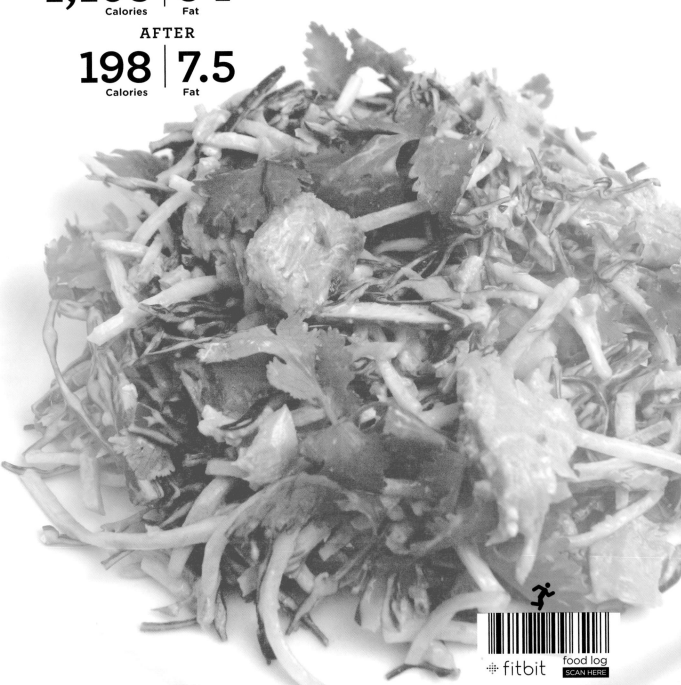

fitbit food log SCAN HERE

SALAD WITH CARROT-GINGER DRESSING

THIS SALAD is the epitome of a dish that's high flavor–low calorie density. The carrots, iceberg lettuce, and cucumber are essentially composed of fiber and water which makes for some serious fill-power. And the metabolism boosting ginger in the fat-free dressing keeps you diggin' in but not missing the typical fat/sugar/salt salad dressing.

Yield	Prep time	Processing time	Calorie Burn	Calories	Net-Calories
1 salad	**approximately 10 minutes**	**approximately 10 minutes**	**34**	**55**	**21**

Ingredients:

½	**large carrot**
1	**(¾-inch) piece fresh ginger, peeled**
1	**tablespoon monk fruit crystals (such as Lakanto Golden Sweetener)**
2	**teaspoons apple cider vinegar**
1	**teaspoon gluten-free reduced-sodium tamari (such as San-J)**
¼	**teaspoon Vietnamese- or Thai-style fish sauce**
¼	**head iceberg lettuce**
¼	**large cucumber, peeled, halved lengthwise, and cut into thin half-moons**
1	**tablespoon finely sliced scallion**
	Lime wedge, for serving

Method:

1. Grate the carrot with a Microplane into a small bowl. Chop the ginger into a fine pulp with a chef's knife and place 1 tablespoon into the bowl with the carrot. Add the monk fruit, vinegar, tamari, and fish sauce to the bowl and mix well.
2. Take the outer leaves off the iceberg, then chop it into bite-sized pieces and place them in a large bowl. Add the cucumber to the bowl with the iceberg.
3. Pour the dressing over the lettuce-cucumber mixture, season with salt and pepper, and mix well. Spoon the mixture onto a plate, top with the scallions, and serve with a lime wedge.

Tip:

Add 2 ounces shredded or diced cooked boneless skinless chicken breast for added protein and about 95 power-packed calories.

Per serving:

55 calories, 0 fat (0.4g sat), 0mg cholesterol, 393mg sodium, 23g carbohydrate, 3.25g fiber, 2.7g protein

Recommended Ready-Made Version:

Annie's Ginger Sesame Dressing
Fat: 8g / Calories: 90 cal

BEFORE

135 | **11**
Calories | Fat

AFTER

55 | **0**
Calories | Fat

fitbit food log
SCAN HERE

COOK YOUR BUTT OFF!

HEART OF PALM AND ESCAROLE SALAD WITH SPICY ORANGES AND AVOCADO

ESCAROLE IS a hearty alkaline salad green to enjoy in the wintertime, the same time oranges are in peak season. This leafy green is high in fiber; 3 ounces provides only about 17 calories but contains 8 percent of the daily recommended intake of fiber. Additionally, it is sturdy enough to get tossed with heartier ingredients, making it a good green to choose for salads you make the night before.

Yield	Prep time	Processing time	Calorie Burn	Calories	Net-Calories
1 salad	approximately 2 minutes	approximately 5 minutes	118	123	5

Ingredients:

¼	head escarole
¾	bottled hot cherry pepper (such as B&G), chopped, plus ¾ teaspoon of its liquid
¼	cup orange sections, cut into large chunks (look in produce for pre-peeled and -cut oranges)
½	cup drained reduced-sodium heart of palm (such as Native Forest), cut into bite-sized pieces
5	fresh basil leaves, lightly chopped
	Kosher salt and freshly ground black pepper
¼	just ripe avocado

Method:

1. Cut any stem and any browned or discolored outer leaves off the escarole and cut the remaining leaves into bite-sized pieces. Wash thoroughly in cold water, then spin dry in a salad spinner and place the dried leaves in a large bowl. Combine the hot pepper and its liquid and the oranges in a small bowl. Add the heart of palm, basil, and orange mixture to the escarole and toss to mix well. Season with salt and black pepper.
2. Slice the avocado into 5 pieces, add to the salad, gently mix together, and spoon onto a salad plate and serve.

Tip:

Add some torn fresh basil leaves for added flavor and only about 1 extra calorie.

Per serving:

123 calories, 6g fat (0.725g sat), 0mg cholesterol, 566mg sodium, 16.5g carbohydrate, 7.8g fiber, 4.25g protein

Recommended Ready-Made Version:

Chop't Salad, with romaine, broccoli, bell peppers, and Spa dressing
Fat: 1.5g / Calories: 155 cal

BEFORE

350 | **22**
Calories | Fat

AFTER

123 | **6**
Calories | Fat

fitbit food log
SCAN HERE

COOK YOUR BUTT OFF!

CAULIFLOWER AND KALE SALAD WITH LEMON

I'VE HARPED already on the virtues of cauliflower. Now I would like to say a few words about kale. Kale is the "new spinach." Yes, I know it looks like a pile of weeds sitting in the produce department, but kale is a miracle green. This veggie is packed with minerals, fiber, antioxidants, and the cancer-fighting phytonutrient sulforaphane. I eat so much kale, I'm surprised my hair hasn't turned green.

Yield	Prep time	Processing time	Calorie Burn	Calories	Net-Calories
1 salad	approximately 5 minutes	approximately 5 minutes	61	43	-18

Ingredients:

1	large leaf Tuscan kale, stem removed, leaf chopped
¼	small head cauliflower, grated
3	cherry tomatoes, halved
1½	teaspoons fresh lemon juice
¾	teaspoon capers, chopped
	Kosher salt and freshly ground black pepper

Method:

1. Place everything in a large bowl, season with salt and pepper, and toss to mix evenly.
2. Spoon the mixture into a salad bowl and serve.

Tips:

• Try adding ½ teaspoon fruity olive oil on a special occasion for a luxurious texture and an added 20 calories per salad.
• Add ½ tablespoon of olive oil to this dish and serve with a simply grilled piece of fish for an added 60 calories and 7g of fat.

Per serving:

43 calories, 0.5g fat (0.0g sat), 0mg cholesterol, 102mg sodium, 9.1g carbohydrate, 3.05g fiber, 2.9g protein

Recommended Ready-Made Version:

Chop't Salad with romaine and kale and tomatoes
Fat: 6g / Calories: 60 cal

BEFORE

215 Calories | **22** Fat

AFTER

43 Calories | **0.5** Fat

fitbit food log
SCAN HERE

LENTIL SALAD WITH SHERRY VINEGAR AND MIREPOIX

SOME FOODS have a reputation for being aphrodisiacs, and lentils are one of them. No wonder this vegetable is a staple of meals in the romance countries such as Italy. Americans, however, aren't too keen on lentils. That's too bad—besides their promised sexual powers, lentils are loaded with fiber, nutrients, and flavor. With 8,000 varieties cultivated around the world, I've never met a lentil I didn't like. Plus, I love the way lentils cook: You don't have to soak them, and they cook fast. I've seasoned the lentils here with mirepoix, a mixture of finely diced sautéed vegetables and herbs.

Yield	Prep time	Processing time	Calorie Burn	Calories	Net-Calories
1 salad	approximately 22 minutes	approximately 2 minutes	121	114	-7

Ingredients:

½	teaspoon fresh thyme leaves
1	tablespoon sherry vinegar
	Kosher salt and freshly ground black pepper
½	cup mirepoix vegetable mix (onion, carrot, celery, root vegetables, etc.)
¼	cup steamed lentils (such as Melissa's)
1	ounce smoked turkey breast (such as Applegate Farms) cut into thin strips
½	head butter lettuce, torn into large pieces

Method:

1. Mix the thyme and sherry vinegar in a small bowl, season generously with pepper, and set aside.
2. Chop the vegetables into small ¼-inch pieces, place them in a microwave-safe bowl, and season with salt and pepper. Cover with parchment paper and microwave on high until they just begin to release some water and steam, 1 to 1½ minutes.
3. Toss the vegetables and lentils in a large bowl with the sherry vinegar mixture and season with salt and pepper. Toss in the turkey and lettuce, spoon onto a plate, and serve.

Tip:

Try adding ½ teaspoon fruity olive oil to the dressing on a special occasion for a luxurious perfume and an added 20 calories per salad.

Per serving:

114 calories, 0.5g fat (0.0g sat), 4.5mg cholesterol, 323mg sodium, 17g carbohydrate, 6g fiber, 12g protein

Recommended Ready-Made Version:

Chop't romaine salad with Spa Balsamic Vinaigrette and smoked turkey
Fat: 4g / Calories: 155 cal

BEFORE

280 | **16**
Calories | Fat

AFTER

114 | **0.5**
Calories | Fat

SALAD AND SOUP RECIPES

fitbit food log
SCAN HERE

FRESH PEA SALAD WITH SMOKED SALMON AND CREAMY HORSERADISH DRESSING

LOTS OF recipes have "secret" ingredients, and the secret here is the delightfully tangy horseradish. Horseradish is actually a root vegetable that has been cultivated since ancient times. At various times in its history, it has been used as an aphrodisiac, a bitter herb for Passover Seders, and a flavorful accompaniment for meat and seafood dishes. Supposedly, horseradish has antibacterial properties, too. I love it and would eat it with everything if I could.

Yield	Prep time	Processing time	Calorie Burn	Calories	Net-Calories
1 salad	approximately 15 minutes	approximately 10 minutes	92	117	25

Ingredients:

Kosher salt

1½ **cups trimmed sugar snap peas**

3 **tablespoons small-diced cucumber**

2 **tablespoons plain soy yogurt (such as Whole Soy & Co.)**

¼ **teaspoon grated lime zest**

2¼ **teaspoons fresh lime juice**

1 **teaspoon prepared horseradish**

1½ **ounces reduced-sodium smoked salmon (such as Trident), cut into ½-inch strips**

¼ **cup fresh cilantro, lightly chopped**

Method:

1. Bring 2 quarts of water to a boil. Add 1 tablespoon of salt, add the peas, and cook until tender but not completely soft, about 30 seconds. Transfer to a bowl of ice water to cool. Drain the peas and pat dry. Set aside.

2. Mix the cucumber, yogurt, lime zest, lime juice, and horseradish in a large bowl and season with salt. Add the peas and mix to coat evenly, then gently fold in the salmon.

3. Transfer the salad to a plate, garnish with the cilantro, and serve.

Tip:

Swap the lime juice with lemon and the cilantro with dill for an equally delicious variation.

Per serving:

117 calories, 2.5g fat (0.02g sat), 7.5mg cholesterol, 239mg sodium, 11.43g carbohydrate, 3g fiber, 14g protein

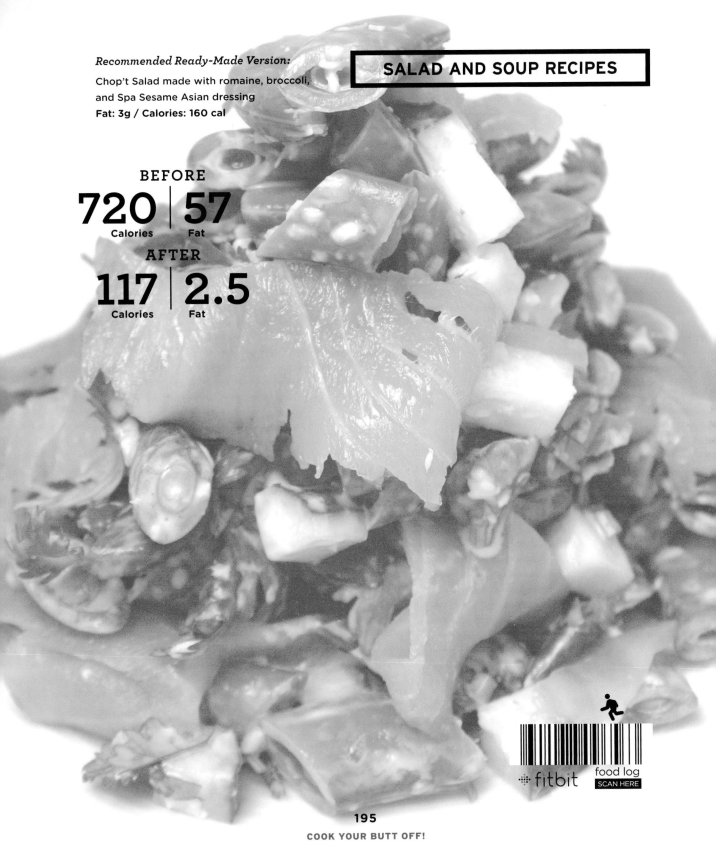

Recommended Ready-Made Version:
Chop't Salad made with romaine, broccoli,
and Spa Sesame Asian dressing
Fat: 3g / Calories: 160 cal

SALAD AND SOUP RECIPES

BEFORE
720 | **57**
Calories | Fat

AFTER
117 | **2.5**
Calories | Fat

fitbit food log
SCAN HERE

GRILLED TURKEY CUTLET WITH PEAR, ARUGULA, AND SPROUT SALAD WITH AVOCADO

THE VEGGIES in this salad are alkaline superstars, meaning the dish is great for cleansing and for weight loss. The combination of flavors dance on the plate: Healthy fat from the avocado, acid and sweetness from the pear, and some heat from the arugula make it happen. And the sprouts? They are loaded with enzymes, nutrients, and fibers. You couldn't ask for a healthier salad!

Yield	Prep time	Processing time	Calorie Burn	Calories	Net-Calories
1 salad	approximately 12 minutes	approximately 15 minutes	123	252	129

Ingredients:

1	**(4-ounce) turkey tender**
	Olive oil cooking spray
	Kosher salt and freshly ground black pepper
1	**small regular pear, or ½ Asian pear**
¼	**teaspoon white wine vinegar**
2	**cups arugula**
½	**cup broccoli sprouts or your favorite sprouts**
⅛	**teaspoon green hot sauce (such as Tabasco Green Jalapeño)**
¼	**just-firm-enough-to-slice avocado, peeled**

Method:

1. Preheat a grill or grill pan to medium-high heat. Place the turkey between two sheets of plastic wrap and pound it until it looks like a cutlet about ¼ inch thick. Spray it with cooking spray, then season with salt and pepper on both sides. Grill to blacken slightly and cook through on both sides, about 2 minutes per side. Transfer to a plate.

2. Grate half of the pear into a bowl, and use half of the puree to top the turkey. Slice the other half of the pear into ¼-inch slices and place them in a bowl with the remaining pear puree, the vinegar, arugula, broccoli sprouts, and Tabasco. Season and place the salad on top of the turkey.

3. Slice the avocado, season the slices with salt, then evenly distribute the slices over the turkey.

Tip:

Serve this dish with a lemon wedge and feel free to add some hot sauce or use your favorite blackening spice on the cutlet before you grill.

Per serving:

252 calories, 8g fat (1.6g sat), 50mg cholesterol, 92.25mg sodium, 14.1g carbohydrate, 4.95g fiber, 29.7g protein

Recommended Ready-Made Version:

Lean Cuisine Honestly Good Pomegranate Chicken
Fat: 9g / Calories: 390 cal

BEFORE

417 | **31.5**
Calories | Fat

AFTER

252 | **8**
Calories | Fat

fitbit food log
SCAN HERE

KIMCHI-CUCUMBER SALAD WITH APPLES AND SHAVED PORK

KIMCHI IS a spicy cabbage side dish that is considered one of the healthiest foods in the world. The fiber in cabbage promotes a healthy digestive system, and kimchi itself unleashes vitamins A, B, and C to work health wonders on the body. Studies show that aged kimchi helps lower blood pressure and cholesterol; it also has disease-fighting antioxidants and digestion-aiding probiotic bacteria similar to those in yogurt.

Yield	Prep time	Processing time	Calorie Burn	Calories	Net-Calories
1 salad	approximately 10 minutes	approximately 10 minutes	69	113	44

Ingredients:

- ¼ cup raw kimchi (such as Rejuvenate), chopped into small pieces with juice
- ¼ cup bean sprouts, lightly chopped
- ¾ cup cucumber, cut into ¼-inch-thick slices
- ¼ cup sliced Granny Smith apples, cut into ¼-inch-thick slices
- ½ teaspoon Thai-style fish sauce
- Kosher salt and freshly ground black pepper
- 1½ ounces roasted pork loin, trimmed of fat, very thinly sliced by your deli
- ¼ cup fresh cilantro
- Lime wedge, for serving

Method:

1. Place the kimchi, bean sprouts, cucumber, apples, and fish sauce into a bowl and mix well to coat. Season with salt and pepper. Fold the slices of pork and place in the middle of a plate.
2. Add the cilantro to the salad and then mound in the center of the pork. Serve with a lime wedge.

Tip:

If you don't eat meat, try substituting ½ cup diced or sliced tofu to this recipe instead.

Per serving:

113 calories, 1.5g fat (.7g sat), 31mg cholesterol, 332mg sodium, 12g carbohydrate, 4g fiber, 13g protein

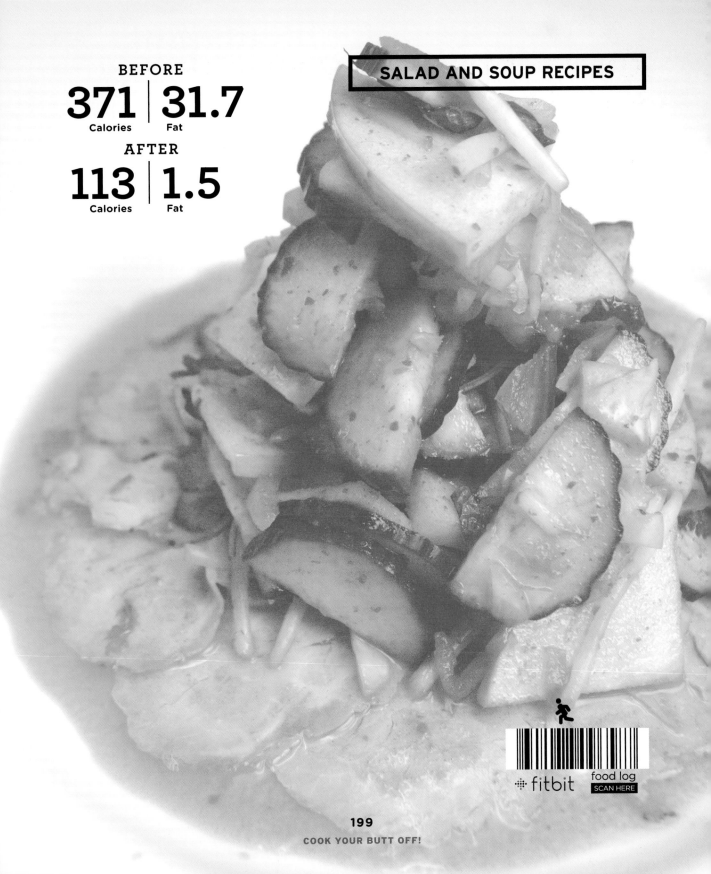

BEFORE

371 | **31.7**
Calories | Fat

AFTER

113 | **1.5**
Calories | Fat

fitbit food log SCAN HERE

CREAM OF MUSHROOM SOUP

I'VE ALWAYS wanted to cook with those dried mushrooms you see in the grocery store—so that's what I did here. When ground to a powder, these little things saturate liquids with all the might of an entire forest of mushrooms! They are the key to this luxurious-tasting classic soup. There's no fattening cream in this soup, either—just high-nutrition soy powder.

Yield	Prep time	Processing time	Calorie Burn	Calories	Net-Calories
8 ounces	approximately 10 minutes	approximately 15 minutes	98	135	37

Ingredients:

1	cup water
½	cup sliced cremini mushrooms
4	dried shiitake mushrooms, ground into a powder
1½	tablespoons soy milk powder (such as Better Than Milk)
2	teaspoons arrowroot powder
	Kosher salt
1½	teaspoons chopped fresh chives

Method:

1. Place ¾ cup of the water into a saucepan with both mushrooms, place it over medium-high heat, and bring to a simmer.
2. Mix the remaining ¼ cup water, soy milk powder, and arrowroot in a small bowl. Once the mushroom mixture comes to a simmer, add the soy-arrowroot mixture to the pan while whisking. Reduce the heat to medium and simmer the soup, stirring, for about one minute. Season with salt.
3. Spoon the soup into a bowl and top with the chopped chives.

Tips:

- If possible, soak the dried and fresh mushrooms in the 1 cup water overnight to maximize the flavor extraction from the mushrooms.
- Add wild mushrooms to this soup or change the dried mushroom variety for a little change from time to time.

Per serving:

135 calories, 1g fat (0g sat, 0g mono, 0g poly), 0mg cholesterol, 88.5mg sodium, 31.7g carbohydrate, 0.45g fiber, 1.75g protein

Recommended Ready-Made Version:

Gluten-free Café Cream of Mushroom
Fat: 6g / Calories: 110 cal

BEFORE

200 | **12**
Calories | Fat

AFTER

135 | **1**
Calories | Fat

fitbit food log SCAN HERE

COOK YOUR BUTT OFF!

HOT-AND-SOUR NOODLE SOUP WITH MUSHROOMS

I LOVE Asian food and have been known to order takeout several times a week. Here's an Asian restaurant standard that you can now enjoy at home. It's so hearty that it feels like a full meal.

Yield	Prep time	Processing time	Calorie Burn	Calories	Net-Calories
12 ounces	approximately 15 minutes	approximately 10 minutes	148	178	30

Ingredients:

Kosher salt

¾ **ounce soy spaghetti (such as Explore Asian)**

1 **cup unsalted fat-free chicken stock (such as Kitchen Basics)**

1 **cup sliced cremini mushrooms**

½ **cup sliced red bell peppers**

¼ **cup sliced onion**

2 **tablespoons coconut aminos (such as Coconut Secret)**

¼ **teaspoon red hot sauce (such as Tabasco Original), plus more as desired**

Method:

1. Bring 2 quarts of water to a boil. Add 1 tablespoon of salt and the spaghetti and stir. Cook for 5 minutes, then drain in a colander. Place the noodles in a bowl and set aside in a warm place.
2. In a large, wide saucepan, place the chicken stock, mushrooms, peppers, and onions, and bring to a boil over high heat. Once boiling, add the noodles, coconut aminos, and hot sauce and season with salt, if needed. Taste and add more hot sauce, if desired.
3. Pour the soup into a bowl and serve.

Tip:

Add ¼ cup fresh cilantro to this soup and a wedge of lime for a little more bang and about 4 calories.

Per serving:

178 calories, 1g fat (0.0g sat), 0mg cholesterol, 685mg sodium, 23g carbohydrate, 6.25g fiber, 21.5g protein

Recommended Ready-Made Version:

Simply Asia Szechwan Hot & Sour Soup
Fat: 5g / Calories: 280 cal

BEFORE

425 | **1**
Calories | Fat

AFTER

178 | **1**
Calories | Fat

fitbit food log
SCAN HERE

CHAPTER 11

Snack Recipes

Autumn Snack Clusters

Crispy Brown Rice and Wasabi Snack

Corn Muffins

Gluten-free Bread Roll

Turkey Jerky

Grilled Sweet Potatoes with Spicy Coconut Nectar

AUTUMN SNACK CLUSTERS

I GOT tired of spending big bucks on PowerBars, so I decided to create my own. It's made from vegetables and a little dried fruit and it tastes just like a PowerBar. I use parsnips here for their naturally sweet flavor and high fiber content. They work so well with sweeter flavors and are a great low calorie density bulking agent. Opt for the larger super hard roots and peel like a carrot. I also added a little cocoa powder and coconut crystals for sweetness. I use beets frequently in my desserts and have done so here as well. The result is a killer snack.

Yield	Prep time	Processing time	Calorie Burn	Calories	Net-Calories
1 snack	approximately 15 minutes	approximately 10 minutes	164	114	-50

Ingredients:

- ¼ cup peeled grated raw beet
- ½ cup peeled grated parsnip
- Kosher salt
- ¼ teaspoon cinnamon
- 1½ tablespoons coconut crystals (such as Coconut Secret)
- 1 packet stevia powder (such as Stevia in the Raw)
- 2 tablespoons crumbled freeze-dried cinnamon-apple crisps (such as Crunchies)
- ¾ teaspoon unsweetened cocoa powder

Method:

1. Preheat the oven to 325°F.
2. Combine the grated vegetables in a large microwave-safe bowl and season lightly with salt. Microwave on high until the vegetables are tender, about 1 minute, then stop, stir, and microwave for 1 minute more.
3. Mix the cinnamon, coconut crystals, and stevia into the vegetables, then form the mixture into 2 even-sized balls. Roll each ball in the crushed apple crisps so they are lightly coated, pressing lightly so the crumbs stick.
4. Place the balls on a wire rack set over a baking sheet and bake until the outsides are dry to the touch and the balls have firmed up a bit, about 10 minutes. Cool the balls in the refrigerator or freezer until cool, then sprinkle with the cocoa powder and serve.

Tips:

- Try adding 1 teaspoon pure vanilla extract to this recipe for added aroma.
- Try adding 1 teaspoon erythritol if you like things a little sweeter.

Per serving:

114 calories, 0.5g fat (0.875g sat), 0mg cholesterol, 120mg sodium, 24.85g carbohydrate, 1.775g fiber, 3.5g protein

Recommended Ready-Made Version:

Two Moms In the Raw organic nut bar, gluten-free
Fat: 9g / Calories: 130 cal

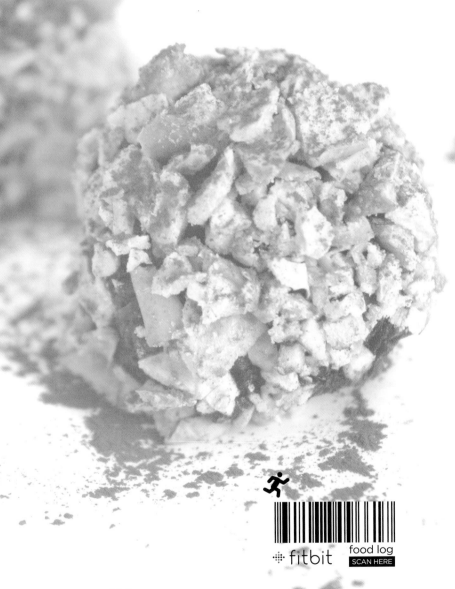

BEFORE

310 | **16**
Calories | Fat

AFTER

114 | **0.5**
Calories | Fat

fitbit food log
SCAN HERE

CRISPY BROWN RICE AND WASABI SNACK

HERE'S MY version of a tasty trail mix. I carry it with me, especially when traveling, for a quick pick-me-up snack. You'll find ingredients here not found in conventional and commercial mixes: nori, a parchment-thin dried seaweed usually found wrapped around sushi; wasabi powder, a spicy Japanese seasoning; and Granny Smith apple chips, a new product I've discovered that adds some necessary sweetness.

Yield	Prep time	Processing time	Calorie Burn	Calories	Net-Calories
1 snack	approximately 10 minutes	approximately 5 minutes	82	95	13

Ingredients:

1   unsalted brown rice cake (such as Lundberg), crumbled into bite-sized pieces
2   sheets nori (2.5g per sheet)
2   tablespoons no-sugar-added Granny Smith apple chips (such as Bare Fruit)
    Olive oil cooking spray
¼   teaspoon natural wasabi powder (such as Eden)
2   teaspoons monk fruit crystals (such as Lakanto Golden Sweetener)
    Kosher salt

Method:

1. Place the crumbled rice cakes into a bowl. Tear 1½ sheets of the nori into 1-inch pieces, then chop the remaining ½ sheet into tiny, powderlike pieces, and add them to the bowl.
2. Place the apple chips on a cutting board and gently smash them with a meat mallet or the side of a chef's knife or cleaver, and add them to the bowl.
3. Spray the mixture for ½ second with cooking spray and sprinkle the wasabi, monk fruit, and salt into the mixture. Stir to coat evenly.
4. Spoon into a snack bowl, and serve.

Tip:

Use this as a base for any snack mix and add what you love. Try hemp hearts, flaxseeds, or toasted shelled pumpkin seeds.

Per serving:

95 calories, 0g fat (0g sat), 0mg cholesterol, 12.5mg sodium, 22.75g carbohydrate, 4.1g fiber, 3g protein

Recommended Ready-Made Version:

Pop Chips
Fat: 4g / Calories: 120 cal

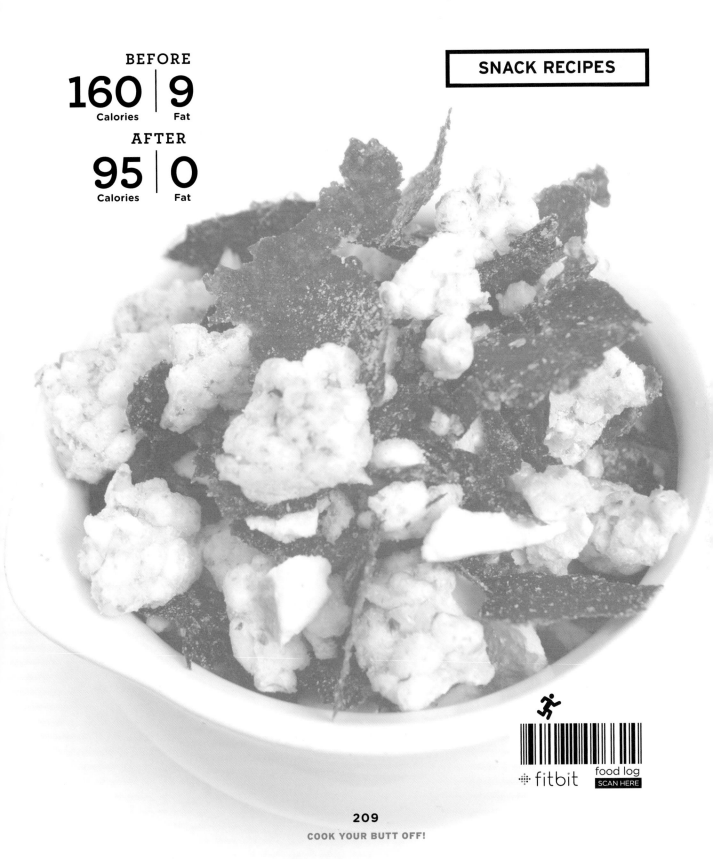

BEFORE

160 | 9
Calories | Fat

AFTER

95 | 0
Calories | Fat

fitbit food log
SCAN HERE

COOK YOUR BUTT OFF!

CORN MUFFINS

HERE IS comfort food from the South—the corn muffin—at its healthiest. They taste delightfully bready, but guess what? They're flourless and gluten-free. I used fresh corn as the "bread" base. That way, I retained micronutrients and highlighted real corn flavor.

Yield	Prep time	Processing time	Calorie Burn	Calories	Net-Calories
2 muffins	approximately 20 minutes	approximately 10 minutes	116	50	-66

Ingredients:

Olive oil cooking spray

2½ **ounces frozen cut corn kernels (such as America's Choice), thawed (about ¼ of a 10-ounce box)**

2 **packets monk fruit powder (such as Monk Fruit in the Raw)**

¼ **teaspoon pure vanilla extract**

Kosher salt

1 **tablespoon gluten-free corn flour (such as Bob's Red Mill)**

2 **tablespoons fresh egg whites (from about 1 large egg)**

Method:

1. Preheat the oven to 350°F. Spray 2 wells of a nonstick cupcake pan with cooking spray.
2. In a blender, combine the corn, monk fruit, and vanilla and blend on high until smooth, about 2 minutes. Season with salt and scrape the mixture into a large bowl. Add the corn flour and mix very well.
3. Whisk the egg whites in a bowl until they form soft peaks. Fold the egg whites into the corn mixture in three additions, being careful not to deflate the whites. Evenly spoon the mixture between the prepared wells of the cupcake pan and bake until cooked through and dry in the middle, 8 to 10 minutes. Serve.

Tips:

- If you like a drier muffin, turn the oven off after the corn muffins are brown, remove them from the cupcake pan, and let them sit in the oven until they are dry.
- You can add 1 teaspoon baking powder to this recipe for a little extra leavening.
- Try adding ⅛ teaspoon ground turmeric to the mixture in the blender if you like a nice yellow muffin.
- Roll the muffins in some monk fruit crystals (such as Lakanto Golden Sweetener) when they come out of the oven for a real sweet touch.

Per serving:

50 calories, 0.5g fat (0g sat), 50mg cholesterol, 50mg sodium, 9.9g carbohydrate, 0.875g fiber, 2.7g protein

Recommended Ready-Made Version:

Pamela's Cornbread and Muffin mix
Fat: 0g / Calories: 80 cal

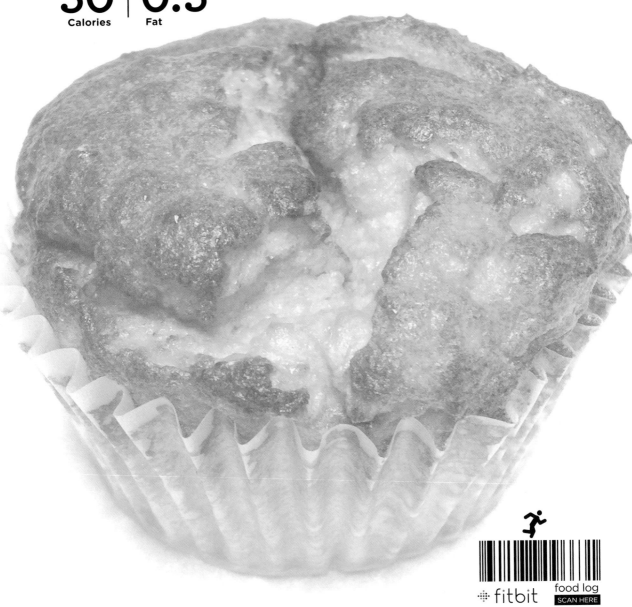

BEFORE

460 | **16**
Calories | Fat

AFTER

50 | **0.5**
Calories | Fat

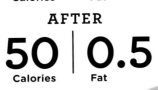

fitbit food log
SCAN HERE

211
COOK YOUR BUTT OFF!

GLUTEN-FREE BREAD ROLL

GLUTEN-FREE bread and rolls are easier and easier to come by nowadays, but finding a low-calorie one is not, let alone one so low in carbs! I've changed all that with this recipe. It can be made in twenty minutes and is very versatile. Experiment with different shapes, cut them in half, and toast the cut sides. This also works great as a guilt free burger bun! Try it with my vegetarian burger!

Yield	Prep time	Processing time	Calorie Burn	Calories	Net-Calories
1 roll	approximately 8 minutes	approximately 20 minutes	189	116	-73

Ingredients:

Olive oil cooking spray

1 large fresh egg white

3 tablespoons cold water

1 tablespoon psyllium husk powder (such as Yerba)

2 tablespoons gluten-free all-purpose flour (such as Glutino)

⅛ teaspoon kosher salt

1 teaspoon coconut spread (such as Olivio)

Method:

1. Preheat the oven to 450°F and place a pizza stone or baking sheet in the oven to heat. Poke holes with a roasting fork in the bottom of a pint-sized microwaveable paper soup container (the kind you get from a takeout soup shop works the best) from the inside out. Spray with cooking spray.

2. In a small bowl, whisk the egg white until it forms soft peaks. Pour the water into a large bowl, add the dry ingredients, mix quickly, then immediately fold in the egg white, being sure not to deflate it too much. Fill the paper cup evenly with the mixture and microwave on high until puffy and just set (just firm to the touch), about 45 seconds.

3. Carefully remove the bun from the container, carefully place it on the preheated pizza stone or baking sheet, and bake until browned and cooked through, 15 to 17 minutes. Remove, let cool on a wire rack, cut in half, and toast in the toaster. Spread the coconut spread on the roll and serve.

Tip:

The key to this recipe is making sure the middle of the bun is dried out enough. Keep the bun in the oven at a lower temperature if it is browned but not dried out enough. Cutting it in half and toasting it works great as well if it is still a little moist inside.

Per serving:

116 calories, 2g fat (0.875g sat), 0mg cholesterol, 383.25mg sodium, 4.75g carbohydrate, 4.5g fiber, 4.48g protein

Recommended Ready-Made Version:

Udi's Classic French Dinner Rolls

Fat: 5g / Calories: 80 cal

BEFORE

350 | **19**
Calories | Fat

AFTER

116 | **2**
Calories | Fat

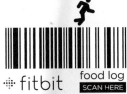

fitbit food log
SCAN HERE

TURKEY JERKY

COMMERCIALLY PRODUCED jerky is normally marinated in seasoning, then dried, dehydrated, or smoked under low heat. It's not too hard to make at home. Normally, you'd use meat strips, but I discovered a killer technique using ground meat instead. You can add any spice you like, but I love the smoky notes from the paprika and a dash of a classic Creole-style blackening spice for a real kick.

Yield	Prep time	Processing time	Calorie Burn	Calories	Net-Calories
1 snack	approximately 10 minutes	approximately 10 minutes	136	45	-91

Ingredients:

1½ ounces extra-lean ground turkey (such as Jennie-O)

⅛ teaspoon kosher salt

½ teaspoon monk fruit crystals (such as Lakanto Golden Sweetener)

¼ teaspoon smoked paprika

⅛ teaspoon blackening spice (such as Phillips)

Method:

1. Combine the turkey, salt, and spices in a bowl and mix together until it forms a smooth paste. You really need to work this hard, so it takes about 2 minutes. On your work surface, lay out a piece of plastic wrap at least 12 inches long. Place the paste in the middle of the plastic sheet and place another piece of plastic wrap over the top. Roll the paste with a rolling pin into a thin sheet about ⅛ inch thick, 7 inches long, and 2 inches wide.

2. Cut the plastic wrap and paste in half lengthwise, then cut each half lengthwise again to form 4 even strips. Remove the top layer of plastic and flip the paste onto a flat microwave-safe plate. Peel off the remaining layer of plastic wrap (the paste should be flat against the plate, without any plastic wrap).

3. Microwave on high for 1 minute, flip the strips of paste, and cook for 30 seconds more. Place a paper towel under the jerky and cook until dried and almost crisp, about 20 seconds more. Transfer to a clean plate, and serve.

Tip:

I like these coming out wafer-thin and crispy, but if you like a leathery jerky, just cook them about 30 seconds less.

Per serving:

45 calories, 0g fat (0.18g sat), 20.6mg cholesterol, 98.75mg sodium, 1g carbohydrate, 0g fiber, 9.75g protein

Recommended Ready-Made Version:

Perky Jerky
Fat: 0g / Calories: 50 cal

BEFORE
116 | **7.25**
Calories | Fat

AFTER
45 | **0**
Calories | Fat

fitbit

food log
SCAN HERE

GRILLED SWEET POTATOES WITH SPICY COCONUT NECTAR

THIS SNACK could almost masquerade as a dessert, it's so delectable, thanks to the use of coconut nectar, my new best friend in the world of natural sweeteners. It can be used as a replacement for the same amount of sugar in recipes. And don't worry: It doesn't taste like coconut. Instead, it has a caramel-like flavor, making it the perfect complement for sweet potatoes.

Yield	Prep time	Processing time	Calorie Burn	Calories	Net-Calories
1 snack/side	approximately 10 minutes	approximately 15 minutes	155	147	-8

Ingredients:

1	small sweet potato, cut into 2 discs ½ inch thick (2½ ounces total)
	Olive oil cooking spray
	Kosher salt and freshly ground black pepper
½	tablespoon coconut nectar (such as Coconut Secret)
½	teaspoon minced red jalapeño
1	tablespoon plain fat-free Greek yogurt (such as Fage 0%)
3	tablespoons hulled dry-roasted pumpkin seeds (such as Eden), chopped

Method:

1. Preheat a grill or grill pan on high heat. Lay the sweet potato discs out, spray them with cooking spray, season with salt and pepper, flip the discs, and repeat.
2. Grill the potatoes until lightly charred on both sides, about 1 minute per side. Place in a microwave-safe bowl, cover with parchment paper, and microwave on high until tender, about 2 minutes. Place the discs on a plate.
3. Mix the coconut nectar with the minced jalapeño and drizzle evenly over the discs. Top with the yogurt and pumpkin seeds and serve.

Per serving:

147 calories, 4g fat (0.62g sat), 0mg cholesterol, 56.25mg sodium, 23g carbohydrate, 2.4g fiber, 4.6g protein

Recommended Ready-Made Version:

Sweet Potato Pop Chips
Fat: 4g / Calories: 120 cal

BEFORE

326.9 | **14.4**
Calories | Fat

AFTER

147 | **4**
Calories | Fat

fitbit food log
SCAN HERE

CHAPTER 12

Dessert Recipes

Chocolate Mousse

Chocolate Mint Thins

Mint Chocolate Chip Flurry

Coconut Clusters

Ice Cream Sandwich

*Sweet Potato and Chocolate Truffle
with Coconut*

No-bake Apple Pie Squares

Carrot Cake

Tartar of Exotic Fruits

Chocolate Cookies

CHOCOLATE MOUSSE

I LOVE chocolate. Luscious, delicious, erotic, simply heavenly chocolate. I believe chocolate is the antidote for depression and bad moods. Everyone gets happy when they eat chocolate. But here's the catch: If you're trying to lose weight or control your weight, chocolate can be one of the first things you crave a few days into a diet. And if you're anything like me, it's hard to work a favorite food like chocolate into my diet, because I'm apt to overindulge. So I figured out a way to take the calories out of one of my favorite chocolate desserts—chocolate mousse. By using the (thankfully) now widely available stevia-sweetened chocolate and good old hard learned French technique, this recipe is a keeper! This baby is darn good, and the recipe saves more than 750 calories per serving over the traditional recipe. Dig in and experience the sheer exhilaration of this heavenly chocolate treat—and you'll love what your scale says.

Yield	Prep time	Processing time	Calorie Burn	Calories	Net-Calories
1 dessert	approximately 10 minutes	approximately 10 minutes	135	121	-14

Ingredients:

½	cup water
19	grams stevia-sweetened chocolate (such as Lily's Original)
43	grams egg whites (about 1 large egg white)
¼	teaspoon pure vanilla extract
1½	level teaspoons egg white powder (4g)
5	grams monk fruit baking mix, about 3 tablespoons (such as Monk Fruit in the Raw)
1	pinch salt

Method:

1. Place the water in a small saucepot over medium heat, place a medium stainless steel mixing bowl over the pot, crumble the chocolate into the bowl, allow to melt and then turn off the heat, about 5 minutes.
2. Place the egg whites, vanilla, egg white powder, monk fruit, and salt into a blender and blend on low until smooth and glossy, about 45 seconds. Scrape the mixture into a medium mixing bowl and whisk until very stiff peaks have formed, about 5 minutes. (I like to use a hand powered mechanical egg-beater.) It should look almost like whipped cream.
3. Remove the melted chocolate from the top of the saucepot and fold in the egg white mixture in three additions while trying to keep the mixture as fluffy as possible. Spoon the mixture into four 4-ounce dishes and place in the refrigerator to chill until set, about 10 minutes. Serve.

Tips:

Once set, cover the bowls and keep in the refrigerator for up to 3 days.

Per serving:

121 calories, 7g fat (6.75g sat), 0mg cholesterol, 150 mg sodium, 15.25g carbohydrate, 6.25g fiber, 6g protein

Recommended Ready-Made Version:

Jello Chocolate Indulgence

Fat: 3g / Calories: 60 cal

BEFORE

909 | **64.5**

Calories | Fat

AFTER

121 | **7**

Calories | Fat

fitbit food log SCAN HERE

CHOCOLATE MINT THINS

I MISS the old Girl Scouts Thin Mints cookies so I wanted to create a natural version of those ubiquitous treats in my own kitchen. I tested my creation out on my cookie-loving friends; the critical reception fell almost unanimously along the lines of "better than the Girl Scout cookie version." Personally, I'd never say that about any Girl Scout cookie, but the recipe is a good one to have.

Yield	Prep time	Processing time	Calorie Burn	Calories	Net-Calories
2 cookies	approximately 10 minutes	approximately 10 minutes	92	55	-37

Ingredients:

2   unsalted brown rice snaps (such as Edward & Sons)
10 grams stevia-sweetened dark chocolate (such as Lily's)
1   drop peppermint pure essential oil (such as Aura Cacia)
2   fresh mint leaves

Method:

1. Lay the rice snaps on a piece of waxed paper on a plate that can fit in your freezer. Put the chocolate in a microwave-safe bowl and microwave on high until the chocolate is soft but not completely liquid then stir in the peppermint oil.

2. Drizzle half of the chocolate evenly over the top of the crackers in a lacy pattern and place a mint leaf on top of each. Drizzle the remaining chocolate over each leaf. Place the plate in the freezer to set the chocolate, 2 to 3 minutes.

3. Remove the plate from the freezer and serve.

Per serving:

55 calories, 4g fat (2.25g sat), 1mg cholesterol, 1.25mg sodium, 8.5g carbohydrate, 0.75g fiber, 3.25g protein

Recommended Ready-Made Version:
Yes! To Cookies Cocoa licious
Fat: 4.5g / Calories: 60 cal

BEFORE

160 | 8

Calories | **Fat**

AFTER

55 | 4

Calories | **Fat**

COOK YOUR BUTT OFF!

MINT CHOCOLATE CHIP FLURRY

I LOVE eating at ice cream parlors every so often. If there's a flurry on the menu, it gets my pick almost every time. But here's the catch: If you're trying to lose or control your weight, a flurry can be a very bad choice. And if you're anything like me, it's hard to work a favorite food like flurries into my diet, because I'm apt to overindulge. So I figured out a way to take the calories out. For starters, I made this flurry practically devoid of sugar by using a gang of no-sugar ingredients. And for years, I've explored the use of natural sugar substitutes—not chemical-laden artificial sweeteners, but the newer crop of more natural alternatives on the market, such as monk fruit, used here for truly natural sweetness. I employed my favorite ice cream taste—mint chocolate chip—to make this flurry a real taste sensation. This will cure any milk shake craving you ever have!

Yield	Prep time	Processing time	Calorie Burn	Calories	Net-Calories
1 (8-ounce) dessert	approximately 10 minutes	approximately 10 minutes	127	119	-8

Ingredients:

- 1   **cup crushed ice**
- ¼   **cup plain fat-free Greek yogurt (such as Fage 0%)**
- 2   **tablespoons fresh mint leaves**
- 2   **tablespoons no-sugar-added dairy-free vanilla frozen dessert (such as So Delicious)**
- ½   **teaspoon pure vanilla extract**
- 2   **packets monk fruit extract (such as Monk Fruit in the Raw)**
- 2   **packets stevia powder (such as Stevia in the Raw)**
-   **Pinch of salt**
- ½   **ounce stevia-sweetened dark chocolate (such as Lily's)**

Method:

1. Smash the ice into a powder in a clean kitchen towel until you have 1 cup total of powdery ice.
2. Place the yogurt, mint, frozen dessert, vanilla extract, monk fruit, stevia, and salt in a hand-slap-chopping gadget and slap until combined. Add the ice and the chocolate and slap until all the ice has been creamed into the mixture.
3. Remove the mixture from the gadget and scrape into an 8-ounce cup.

Tips:

- Add 1 tablespoon unsweetened cocoa powder for an added chocolate layer for just 10 additional calories.
- Add 1 scoop of egg white protein (such as Jay Robb) for an extra 25g of protein and 110 calories per serving.
- You can use a blender if you are feeling lazy!

Per serving:

119 calories, 7 g fat (3.3g sat), 0mg cholesterol, 50mg sodium, 15g carbohydrate, 7g fiber, 7g protein

Recommended Ready-Made Version:
So Delicious No-Sugar-Added Mint Chip
Fat: 11g / Calories: 120 cal

BEFORE
548 | 28
Calories | Fat

AFTER
119 | 7
Calories | Fat

fitbit food log
SCAN HERE

COCONUT CLUSTERS

I LOVE this cookie because it resembles a coconut macaroon. Okay, it doesn't taste exactly like one but if you eat these instead, your waistline (and arteries) will thank you! It's made with parsnips, which are naturally sweet. Parsnips are a good source of dietary fiber, and a single serving of parsnips packs loads of antioxidant vitamin C and the heart-healthy B vitamin folate. Once it's coated with the coconut frozen dessert, it seems to fit right at home as a cookie ingredient.

Yield	Prep time	Processing time	Calorie Burn	Calories	Net-Calories
2 clusters	approximately 10 minutes	approximately 10 minutes	101	91	-10

Ingredients:

¼ heaping cup peeled grated parsnips (grated on large holes of a box grater)

1 tablespoon no-sugar-added vanilla coconut frozen dessert (such as So Delicious)

1 packet stevia powder (such as Stevia in the Raw)

1 teaspoon erythritol (such as Wholesome Sweeteners)

1½ teaspoons egg white powder (such as Deb El Just Whites)

Pinch of salt

¼ ounce stevia-sweetened chocolate (such as Lily's)

Method:

1. Preheat the oven to 350°F. Sprinkle the grated parsnip in an even layer over a nonstick baking sheet and bake until the parsnip shreds are almost tender but still toothsome (like shredded coconut) and slightly dry, 2 to 3 minutes. Remove from the oven and reduce the oven temperature to 300°F.

2. In a bowl, combine the coconut dessert, stevia, erythritol, egg white powder, and salt and mix well. Add the cooked parsnips to the bowl and toss to coat evenly. Form 2 even-sized, loosely packed cookie-like clusters on the baking sheet and return to the oven to bake until dried and the edges of the parsnips have just begun to brown, 5 to 7 minutes.

3. Remove the clusters gently, transfer to a plate, and cool completely in the refrigerator. Place the chocolate in a small microwave-safe bowl and cook on high until it has just melted, about 20 seconds. Drizzle the chocolate evenly over each cluster and let set in the refrigerator, about 2 minutes. Serve.

Tips:

Try adding 1 teaspoon of unsweetened, reduced-fat coconut flakes or add 1 teaspoon of coconut manna for an added coconut boost and only about 30 calories.

Per serving:

91 calories, 5g fat (0.875g sat), 0mg cholesterol, 45mg sodium, 14g carbohydrate, 5.5g fiber, 3.25g protein

Recommended Ready-Made Version:

Lily's Coconut Dark Chocolate
Fat: 15g / Calories: 170 cal

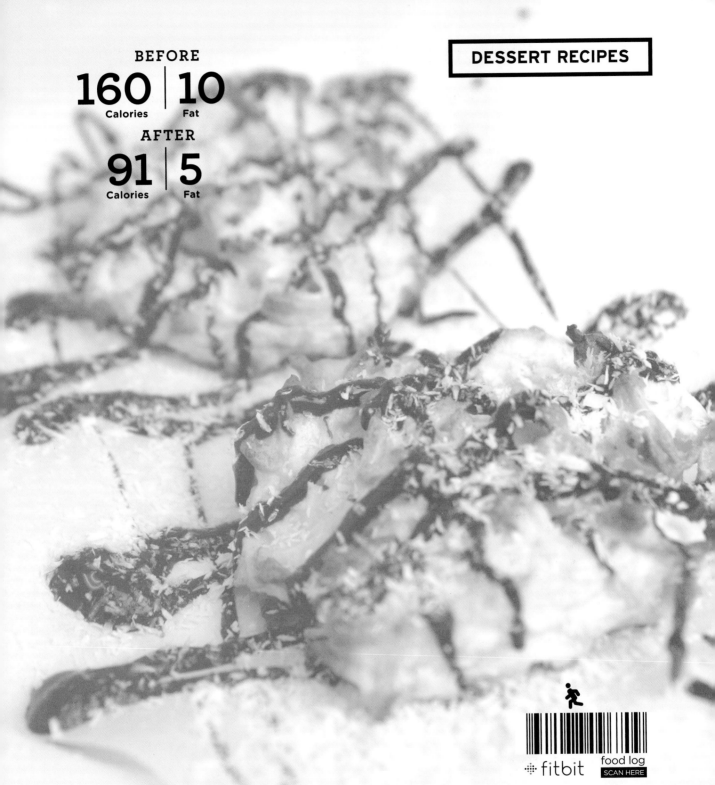

BEFORE

160 | 10
Calories | Fat

AFTER

91 | 5
Calories | Fat

fitbit **food log** SCAN HERE

Shown with unsweetened, reduced-fat coconut flakes

ICE CREAM SANDWICH

THERE ARE various stories as to how this classic ice cream treat came to be, so no one really knows the real scoop. What we do know is that the ice cream sandwich is the number one ice cream product in the marketplace. It's surprisingly easy to make at home, and you'll learn how here. Feel free to substitute different flavors of no-sugar-added coconut milk frozen desserts to suit your preferences. And by the way, this interpretation is lower in calories than the reduced-calorie ice cream sandwiches in the supermarket freezer section (no preservatives added, either!). Another plus: This dessert can last in the freezer for days.

Yield	Prep time	Processing time	Calorie Burn	Calories	Net-Calories
1 sandwich	approximately 5 minutes	approximately 10 minutes	86	95	9

Ingredients:

1   unsalted brown rice thin cake (such as Suzie's)
6   grams stevia-sweetened dark chocolate (such as Lily's)
3   tablespoons dairy-free no-sugar-added vanilla frozen dessert (such as So Delicious)

Method:

1. Place a bowl in the freezer to chill.
2. Lay the rice thin on a cutting board and cut it in half with a sharp knife. Place 3 grams of chocolate on each half and transfer to a microwave-safe plate. Microwave on high until the chocolate has softened but is not fully melted, about 20 seconds. Spread the chocolate over each thin to coat it entirely and place the plate in the freezer to cool until the chocolate has re-hardened, 2 to 3 minutes.
3. Place the frozen dessert in the chilled bowl and mash it with a sturdy fork to form a softer, just-spreadable product. Place the frozen dessert on the noncoated side of one of the rice thins, top with another rice thin, uncoated side facing the ice cream, and gently press to spread the frozen dessert to the edges. Place back in the freezer until ready to serve.

Tip:

Place the ice cream into a chilled mortar and use the pestle to mash any ingredient you want inside—mint leaves, frozen cherries, and so forth.

Per serving:

95 calories, 5g fat (2.25g sat), 0.6mg cholesterol, 2.625mg sodium, 13.425g carbohydrate, 2.325g fiber, 0.925g protein

Recommended Ready-Made Version:

So Delicious Vanilla Coconut Mini
Fat: 3.5g / Calories: 100 cal

BEFORE

230 | 7

Calories | Fat

AFTER

95 | 5

Calories | Fat

DESSERT RECIPES

fitbit food log SCAN HERE

SWEET POTATO AND CHOCOLATE TRUFFLE WITH COCONUT

A CHOCOLATE truffle is a type of candy, traditionally made with a gooey sweet center coated in icing or chopped nuts and formed into a spherical or conical shape. In this version, my center is formed from sweet potatoes, cocoa, and monk fruit and coated with coconut. I think you'll agree: It's yummy.

Yield	Prep time	Processing time	Calorie Burn	Calories	Net-Calories
2 truffles	approximately 2 minutes	approximately 10 minutes	180	59	-121

Ingredients:

- ½ cup peeled grated sweet potatoes
- ⅛ teaspoon pure vanilla extract
- 2½ teaspoons unsweetened cocoa powder
- 2 packets monk fruit powder (such as Monk Fruit in the Raw)
- 1 packet stevia extract (such as Stevia in the Raw)
- ½ teaspoon unrefined coconut oil (such as Spectrum)
- Kosher salt
- 2¼ teaspoons unsweetened reduced-fat shredded coconut (such as Let's Do Organic)
- ½ teaspoon erythritol

Method:

1. Place the sweet potatoes in a microwave-safe bowl, cover with a microwave-safe plate, and microwave on high until the potatoes are just about tender, 2 to 3 minutes. Remove from the microwave and add the vanilla, cocoa powder, monk fruit, stevia, and coconut oil. Stir well, season with salt, and place in the freezer to cool, about 4 minutes.
2. Place the coconut and erythritol in a shallow bowl.
3. Form the sweet potato mixture into 2 loosely packed equal-sized balls and roll them between your hands to tightly pack them. Place each ball in the erythritol and coconut mixture and press the mixture into the sweet potato center, covering the outside of each ball completely. Serve.

Per serving:

59 calories, 5g fat (2.4g sat), 0mg cholesterol, 45.3mg sodium, 8.3g carbohydrate, 2g fiber, 1g protein

Tip:

Keep chilled in an airtight container if you're not eating them right away.

Recommended Ready-Made Version:

Lily's Stevia Dark Sweetened Coconut Chocolate
Fat: 15g / Calories: 170 cal

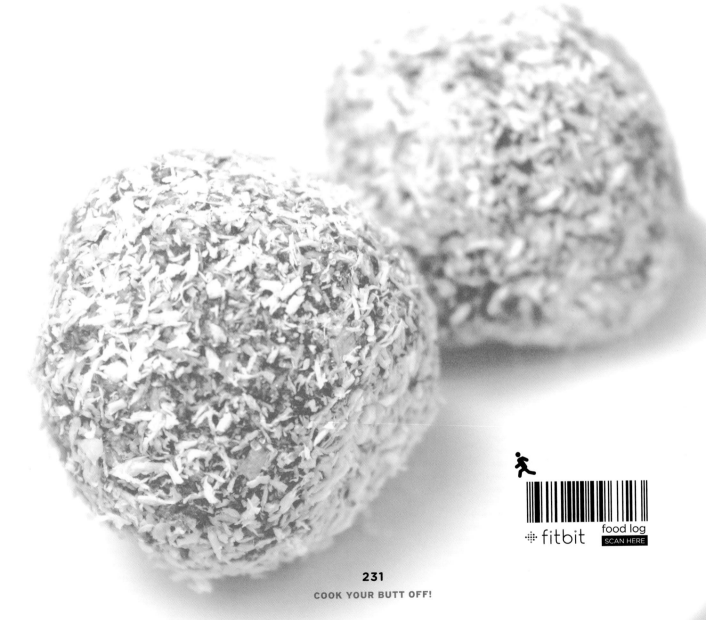

BEFORE

210 | **13**
Calories | Fat

AFTER

59 | **5**
Calories | Fat

fitbit food log
SCAN HERE

NO-BAKE APPLE PIE SQUARES

I, FOR ONE, love apple pie, especially with a dollop or two of real whipped cream. But, like most desserts, it has a lot of sugar and fat, and I don't recommend you eat a whole piece. Instead, I recommend that you try this apple recipe. It has only 94 calories a serving, compared to traditional apple pie at nearly 280 calories a wedge (so you may be able to get away with enjoying two pieces!).

Yield	Prep time	Processing time	Calorie Burn	Calories	Net-Calories
1 dessert	approximately 10 minutes	approximately 15 minutes	130	94	-36

Ingredients:

¼	cup water
¼	cup peeled, grated apples (choose your favorite—I love Empire or Pink Lady apples)
¼	teaspoon plus ⅛ teaspoon fresh lemon juice
1	tablespoon coconut crystals (such as Coconut Secret)
¼	teaspoon ground cinnamon
1	teaspoon pectin (such as Pomona's)
2	packets stevia extract (such as Stevia in the Raw)
2	pieces unsalted brown rice thin cakes (such as Suzie's)

Method:

1. Place the water, apples, lemon juice, coconut, and cinnamon in a large microwave-safe bowl. Cover with a microwave-safe plate or waxed paper and microwave on high until the mixture has come to a boil, about 3 minutes. Remove the bowl from the microwave.
2. In a small bowl, stir together the pectin and stevia and then add it to the hot apple mixture slowly while whisking, until dissolved. Scrape the sides of the bowl, cover, and microwave on high until boiling and thickened, about 30 seconds. Transfer the apple mixture to a stainless-steel bowl and set it over another bowl of ice to chill the mixture completely. It will get much tighter as it cools.
3. Lay a rice thin down on a clean surface, dollop the apple mixture on top, top with a plain rice thin, and serve.

Tip:

I like to keep the mixture right in the bowl and use the crackers as a dip when I need a soul-satisfying sweet snack.

Per serving:

94 calories, 0 fat (0g sat), .25mg cholesterol, 100.5mg sodium, 22.75g carbohydrate, 4.21g fiber, 0.7g protein

Recommended Ready-Made Version:

Apple Pie Quest Bar
Fat: 5g / Calories: 170 cal

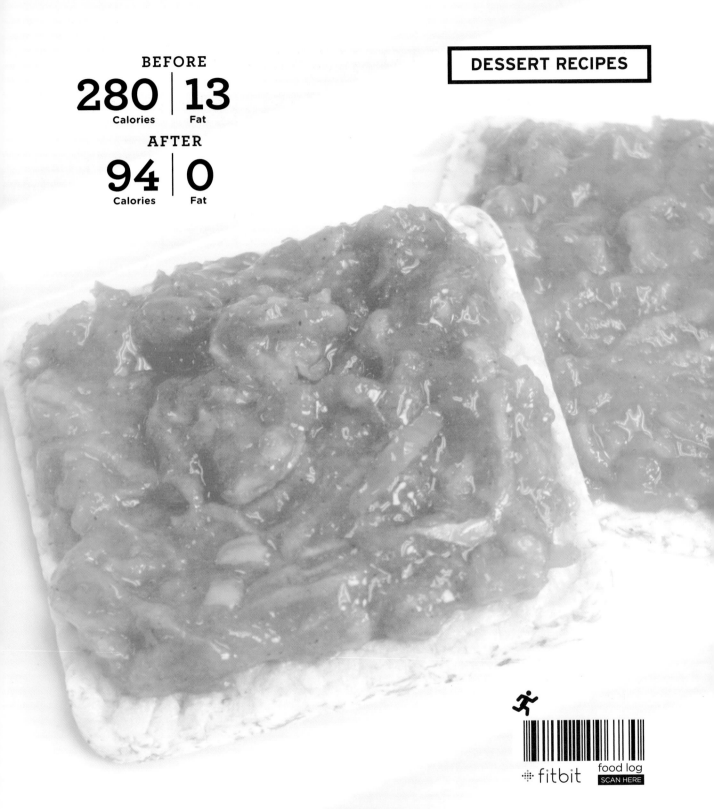

BEFORE

280 | **13**
Calories | Fat

AFTER

94 | **0**
Calories | Fat

DESSERT RECIPES

fitbit food log
SCAN HERE

CARROT CAKE

THERE'S NO denying it—when people go gluten-free, they think they might have to give up cake. But do they? No, and this carrot cake is proof. Carrot cake had always captured my heart—but for dieting, it plays hard to get. I wanted to come up with a magical adaptation that would capture the richness of its original, minus the butter, sugar, and gluten. I did it with some simple but tasty substitutions you can try with just about any baked good.

Yield	Prep time	Processing time	Calorie Burn	Calories	Net-Calories
1 dessert	approximately 3 minutes	approximately 20 minutes	147	90	-57

Ingredients:

Olive oil cooking spray

¼ cup finely grated carrots

½ large fresh egg white

1 tablespoon cold water

¼ teaspoon pure vanilla extract

1½ teaspoons psyllium husk powder (such as Yerba)

2¼ teaspoons gluten-free all-purpose flour (such as Glutino)

¼ teaspoon ground cinnamon

1½ teaspoons monk fruit crystals (such as Lakanto Golden Sweetener)

½ packet stevia (such as Stevia in the Raw)

⅛ teaspoon kosher salt

1 tablespoon no-sugar-added frozen coconut dessert (such as So Delicious Vanilla Bean)

Freshly grated nutmeg, to garnish

Method:

1. Preheat the oven to 350°F. Poke holes with a roasting fork in the bottom of an 8-ounce microwaveable paper cup (a plain paper drinking cup, white, with no liner) from the inside out. Spray with cooking spray.

2. Spread the carrots on a nonstick baking sheet and bake until dried but not browned, 3 to 5 minutes. Cool in the freezer. Leave the oven on.

3. In a bowl, whisk the egg white until it forms soft peaks. Pour the water and vanilla into a large bowl, add the dry ingredients, mix quickly, add the carrots, and then immediately fold in the egg white, being sure not to deflate it too much. Fill the container evenly with the mixture and microwave on high until it is puffy and just set, about 40 seconds.

4. Carefully remove the cake from the container, place it in the oven, and bake until the sides are browned and the cake is cooked through, 3 to 5 minutes. Place the cake on a plate and using a tablespoon measure, place a scoop of the frozen dessert on the cake and garnish with nutmeg.

Tip:

The key to this recipe is making sure the middle of the cake is dried out enough. Keep the cake in the oven at a lower temperature if it is browned but not dried out enough.

Per serving:

90 calories, 1g fat (0g sat), 0mg cholesterol, 267mg sodium,
9.5g carbohydrate, 6.5g fiber, 2.84g protein

Recommended Ready-Made Version:

Go Raw 100% Organic Super Cookies Carrot Cake
Fat: 7g / Calories: 150 cal

BEFORE

321 | 15
Calories | Fat

AFTER

90 | 1
Calories | Fat

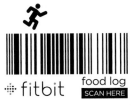

fitbit food log
SCAN HERE

TARTAR OF EXOTIC FRUITS

HERE'S A dish that will transport you to the islands, if only by taste. It combines tropical fruits with the zippy flavors of lime, cilantro, and jalapeño, touched with coconut milk. Hmmm, I can almost feel that island breeze.

	Yield	Prep time	Processing time	Calorie Burn	Calories	Net-Calories
	1 dessert	approximately 4 minutes	approximately 18 minutes	158	79	-79

Ingredients:

1	small ripe mango (1½ ounces of flesh needed)
1	small ripe papaya (1½ ounces of flesh needed)
¼	bunch fresh cilantro stems
¼	teaspoon grated lime zest
½	teaspoon fresh lime juice
½	packet monk fruit powder (such as Monk Fruit in the Raw)
1½	tablespoons lite coconut milk (such as Thai Kitchen)
½	packet stevia powder (such as Stevia in the Raw)
	Tiny pinch of salt
3	grams freeze-dried pineapple (such as Nature's All)

Method:

1. Peel the mango and papaya and weigh out 1½ ounces each fruit. Lightly chop the fruit into small fork-sized pieces and place them in a bowl. Add the cilantro stems, lime zest, half of the lime juice, and the monk fruit. Gently mix together and mound the fruit into a bowl.
2. Mix the remaining lime juice, coconut milk, stevia, and salt in a separate small bowl. Pour the milk over the bowl of fruit, crumble the pineapple evenly over the top, and serve.

Tip:

Add ⅛ teaspoon minced jalapeño for a little zip—trust me, it's great!!!

Per serving:

79 calories, 1.5g fat (1.15g sat), 0mg cholesterol, 20mg sodium, 16.25g carbohydrate, 2g fiber, 0.7g protein

Recommended Ready-Made Version:

Del Monte No-Sugar-Added Assorted Flavor Fruit Cup
Calories: 25 / Fat 0g

BEFORE
300 | **21**
Calories | Fat

AFTER
79 | **1.5**
Calories | Fat

fitbit food log SCAN HERE

COOK YOUR BUTT OFF!

CHOCOLATE COOKIES

A GOOD healthy chocolate cookie recipe is essential when controlling your sweet tooth. A no added sugar, low fat chocolate cookie with 4 grams of protein is just amazing!

Yield	Prep time	Processing time	Calorie Burn	Calories	Net-Calories
6 cookies	**approximately 15 minutes**	**approximately 15 minutes**	**122**	**47**	**-75**

Ingredients:

¼   **cup unsweetened cocoa powder**

¼   **cup erythritol (such as Wholesome Sweeteners)**

5   **packets stevia extract powder (such as Stevia in the Raw)**

¼   **teaspoon salt**

1   **tablespoon unrefined coconut oil, at room temperature**

¼   **cup textured vegetable protein**

2   **freshly separated egg whites**

¼   **teaspoon pure vanilla extract**

Method:

1. Preheat the oven to 350°F. Mix the cocoa, sweeteners, and salt in a mixing bowl. Add the coconut oil and whisk very hard with a whisk until you have a smooth paste, about 1 minute. Place the TVP in between parchment paper and using a meat mallet, crush into pieces about half its original size.

2. Using a clean whisk, whip the egg whites and vanilla extract until soft peaks have formed. Add half the amount of TVP to the cocoa mixture, begin mixing in the egg whites until the cocoa mixture is loose, and then fold in the remaining egg whites and TVP.

3. Place 6 even clumps of the mixture onto a nonstick cookie sheet and place in the oven. Cook until the cookies have visibly risen, allow to cook for 3 minutes, then turn the heat down to 300°F and cook until the cookies have dried out and seem cakey to the touch.

4. Remove the cookies and place on a wire rack to cool. Once they have cooled they will be crisp and ready to serve.

Tips:

Melt some sugar free, naturally sweetened dark chocolate (such as Lily's) and drizzle over the cookies before cooling for an added treat!

Per serving (per cookie):

47 calories, 3g fat (2.28g sat), 0mg cholesterol, 120mg sodium, 15.3g carbohydrate, 1.86g fiber, 3.9g protein

Recommended Ready-Made Version:

Yes! To Cookies Cocoa Licious
Fat: 4.5 g / Calories: 60 cal

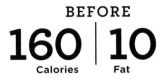

BEFORE
160 | **10**
Calories | Fat

AFTER
47 | **3**
Calories | Fat
(per cookie)

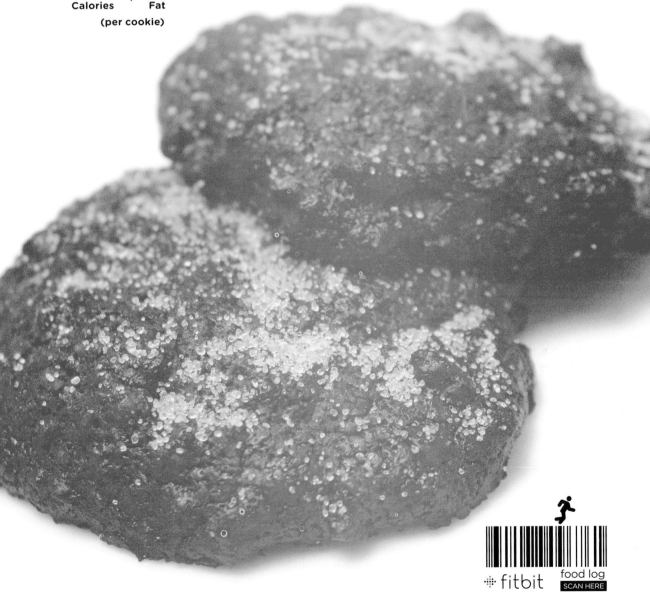

fitbit food log SCAN HERE

RESOURCES

www.calorieking.com

Excellent source for calorie counts for a wide variety of foods.

www.myfitnesspal.com

Estimated calorie burns for many different physical activities.

www.mayoclinic.com

Great health information from the Mayo Clinic, a trusted source.

www.webmd.com

Lots more great health information from another trusted authority.

www.hsph.harvard.edu/nutritionsource/

The Harvard School of Public Health, good info on a wide variety of nutrition and weight control topics.

www.pubmed.com

A superb government website that indexes a huge number of research papers on health, fitness, nutrition, and weight loss published in peer-reviewed medical and scientific journals. An excellent filter to bypass the oceans of bad information on the Internet and get to the good stuff.

www.choosemyplate.gov/SuperTracker/

Exactly how many calories you should consume to maintain or lose weight can be a complex subject that can depend on your sex, height, weight, body type, and activity level. This is a good, free U.S. government website for calculating your personalized daily calorie target that takes these variables into account, with a program called the SuperTracker. Let's say you're a thirty-five-year-old American woman who is around the average height and weight, 5 feet 4 inches and 163 pounds; is not breastfeeding or pregnant, and does an average of less than thirty minutes per day of moderate-intensity physical activity. The bad news: According to the BMI chart, you're overweight, because you have a 28 BMI. The good news: You've got an estimated "magic number" to shoot for. According to the SuperTracker, on average, to move down to a healthy weight, you should eat **1,800 calories a day**. If you wanted to get to a healthy weight faster, you would eat even fewer calories a day and add in physical activity, or do some combination of both.

If you're a man of thirty-five who is around the average height and weight, 5 feet 9 inches and 190 pounds, and does an average of less than thirty minutes per day of moderate-intensity physical activity, the bad news is that according to the BMI chart, you're overweight because you also have a 28 BMI. The good news: According to the SuperTracker, on average, to move down to a healthy weight, you should eat 2,400 calories a day. If you wanted to get to a healthy weight faster, you would eat even fewer calories a day and add in physical activity, or do some combination of both.

Additional notes on weight loss: Kevin D. Hall, PhD, of the National Institutes of Health argued in a 2008 paper in the *International Journal of Obesity* ("What is the Required Energy [calorie] Deficit per unit Weight Loss?") that while the "3500 calorie deficit = 1 pound of weight loss" formula could be accurate for some people, "a larger cumulative energy deficit [calorie deficit] is required per unit weight loss for people with greater initial body fat," which may explain "why men can lose more weight than women for a given energy deficit [calorie deficit] since women typically have more body fat than men of similar body weight." In a 2011 paper in *The Lancet* ("Quantifying the Effect of Energy Imbalance on Body Weight Change"), Hall and his colleagues presented an online Body Weight Simulator tool you may want to check out with your doctor. The simulator estimates body weight changes over time with different levels of calories and physical activity. Find the simulator at bwsimulator.niddk.nih.gov/.

Also, the authors of a 2008 article in the journal *Obesity*, "Successful Weight Loss Maintenance in Relation to Method of Weight Loss," pointed out that the definition of a very-low-calorie diet is arbitrary and can vary depending on the person: "A 700 kcal/d [calories per day] diet, for example, would induce a relatively modest energy [calorie] deficit in a short, sedentary woman with a resting energy [calorie] expenditure (REE) of 1100 kcal/d. In contrast, a 1200 kcal/d diet would induce a substantial energy [calorie] deficit in a tall man with an REE of 2500 kcal/d. The man would seem to have a greater risk of adverse metabolic effects . . . even though technically he was prescribed an LCD and the woman a VLCD. Thus, an alternative definition of a VLCD is a diet that provides <50% of an individual's predicted REE."

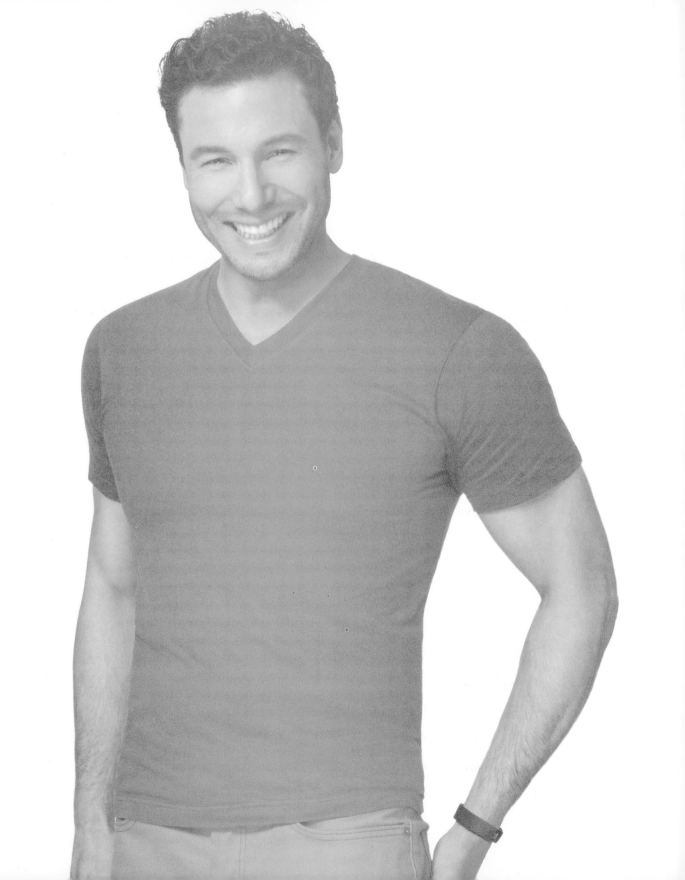

REFERENCES

Cunningham, S. A., et al. 2014. "Incidence of childhood obesity in the United States." *New England Journal of Medicine* 370: 403–411.

Descalzo, A. M., et al. 2005. "Influence of pasture or grain-based diets supplemented with vitamin E on antioxidant/oxidative balance of Argentine beef." *Meat Science* 70: 35–44.

Farrell, R. J., and Ciarán, P. K. 2002. "Celiac Sprue." *New England Journal of Medicine* 346: 180–188.

Holtcamp, W. 2012. "Obesogens: An Environmental Link to Obesity." *Environmental Health Perspectives* 120: a62–a68.

Jonsson, T., et al. 2005. "Agrarian diet and diseases of affluence—do evolutionary novel dietary lectins cause leptin resistance?" *BMC Endocrine Disorders* 5: 10.

Ley, R. E., et al. 2006. "Microbial ecology: human gut microbes associated with obesity." *Nature* 444: 1022–1023.

Schwalfenberg, G. K. 2013. "The alkaline diet: is there evidence that an alkaline pH diet benefits health?" *Journal of Environmental and Public Health* 2012: 1–7.

Sia, J., et al. 2010. "Cyclic voltammetric analysis of antioxidant activity in cane sugars and palm sugars from Southeast Asia." *Food Chemistry* 118: 840–846.

Soares, F. L., et al. 2013. "Gluten-free diet reduces adiposity, inflammation and insulin resistance associated with the induction of PPAR-alpha and PPAR-gamma expression." *Journal of Nutritional Biochemistry* 24: 1,105–1,111.

Welch, A. A., et al. 2013. "A higher alkaline dietary load is associated with greater indexes of skeletal muscle mass in women." *Osteoporosis International* 24: 1899–1908.

Youngman, L. D., and Campbell, T. C. 1991. "High protein intake promotes the growth of hepatic preneoplastic foci in Fischer #344 rats: evidence that early remodeled foci retain the potential for future growth." *Journal of Nutrition* 121: 1454–1461.

INDEX

W

X

Y

Z

ABOUT
ROCCO DISPIRITO

ROCCO DISPIRITO is an award winning chef and author of ten highly-acclaimed cookbooks, including #1 *New York Times* best seller *The Pound A Day Diet*. A cultural phenomenon that revolutionizes dieting, *The Pound A Day Diet* is designed to help you lose up to five pounds every five days—without frustrating plateaus—all while enjoying your favorite foods. This multi-talented chef is also the author of the #1 *New York Times* best-selling series *Now Eat This!* which features healthy makeovers of America's favorite comfort foods.

This entrepreneurial chef recently launched a technologically advanced, fresh food delivery program that combines the luxury of a private chef experience with the convenience of nutritious, flavorful meals. Celebrity clients include Whoopi Goldberg, Sherri Shepherd, Kris Jenner and Paul Stanley, among many others. These stars have experienced safe, rapid weight loss on this program which also features daily personal coaching from Rocco himself.

Rocco joined the hit primetime series *Extreme Weight Loss* on ABC, which premiered on May 27, 2014. Now in its fourth season, this unique, non-competitive series about weight-loss documents the unprecedented 365-day transformation of courageous, obese participants. During their journey, Rocco helps participants learn how to lose a pound a day.

Among his many popular TV series over the years, Rocco has also recently starred in shows such as *Restaurant Divided* on Food Network in the fall of 2013 and *Now Eat This! with Rocco DiSpirito*, a weekly, nationally-syndicated series in 2012. His reality series *Rocco's Dinner Party* aired during the summer of 2011 on Bravo.

In 2012 Rocco founded Savory Place Media, his production house. Its first project *Now Eat This! Italy* for AOL Originals became an instant Top 10 series on AOL, garnering millions of views.

Rocco is also the founder of the *Now Eat This!* food truck, which features meals created from his wildly successful series of cookbooks of the same name.

This generous chef actively dedicates his time to charitable causes. He serves as a HealthCorps Ambassador, wherein he visits schools around the country to educate and excite students about healthy eating. Additionally, in the aftermath of Hurricane Sandy, Rocco served more than 350,000 hot meals to storm victims and volunteers through his *Now Eat This!* food truck.

Rocco began his culinary studies at the Culinary Institute of America and by 20 was working in the kitchens of legendary chefs around the globe. He was voted *Food & Wine* magazine's "Best New Chef," named *People* magazine's "Sexiest Chef Alive" and was the first chef to appear on *Gourmet* magazine's cover as "America's Most Exciting Young Chef." His 3-Star restaurant Union Pacific was a New York City culinary landmark for many years.

Rocco is a frequent guest on *Good Morning America, Rachael Ray, The Talk, The Dr. Oz Show, The View*, among many other programs. When he is not cooking and spreading a healthy eating message, he enjoys bicycling and participating in triathlons.